Workbook for

Comprehensive Radiographic Pathology

Eighth Edition

Workbook for

Comprehensive Radiographic Pathology

Eighth Edition

Ronald L. Eisenberg, MD, JD, FACR
Professor of Radiology
Harvard Medical School
Staff Radiologist
Beth Israel Deaconess Medical Center
Boston, Massachusetts

Editor

Tammy Curtis, Ph.D., RT(R)(CT)(CHES)
Professor, Director
Bachelor of Science in Radiologic Sciences Program
Northwestern State University
Shreveport, Louisiana

ELSEVIER

Elsevier
3251 Riverport Lane
St. Louis, Missouri 63043

WORKBOOK FOR
COMPREHENSIVE RADIOGRAPHIC PATHOLOGY,
EIGHTH EDITION

ISBN: 978-0-443-24975-4

Notice

Practitioners and researchers must always rely on their own experience and knowledge in evaluating and using any information, methods, compounds or experiments described herein. Because of rapid advances in the medical sciences, in particular, independent verification of diagnoses and drug dosages should be made. To the fullest extent of the law, no responsibility is assumed by Elsevier, authors, editors or contributors for any injury and/or damage to persons or property as a matter of products liability, negligence or otherwise, or from any use or operation of any methods, products, instructions, or ideas contained in the material herein.

Previous edition copyrighted 2021

Content Strategist: Meg Benson
Content Development Specialist: Dominque McPherson
Publishing Services Manager: Deepthi Unni
Senior Project Manager: Kamatchi Madhavan
Design Direction: Gopal Venkatraman

Printed in India

Last digit is the print number: 9 8 7 6 5 4 3 2 1

Contents

1 Introduction to Pathology

OBJECTIVES

In addition to the objectives listed at the beginning of Chapter 1 in the textbook, the user should be able to:

1. Classify the more common disease categories described in this chapter:
   - edema
   - hemorrhage
   - hereditary
   - iatrogenic
   - idiopathic
   - infarction
   - inflammation
   - ischemia
   - neoplasia

2. Define or describe the following terms from this chapter:
   - abscess
   - acquired immunodeficiency syndrome (AIDS)
   - antibodies
   - antigens
   - aplasia
   - asymptomatic
   - atrophy
   - bacteremia
   - benign
   - carcinoma
   - diagnosis
   - dysplasia
   - epidemiology
   - etiology
   - exudate
   - grading
   - granulomatous
   - immunity
   - hematoma
   - hyperemia
   - hypertrophy
   - hypoplasia
   - malignant
   - morbidity
   - mortality
   - nosocomial
   - pathology
   - permeable
   - prognosis
   - pyogenic
   - scar
   - seeding
   - staging
   - standard precautions
   - toxins
   - transudate
   - transmission-based precautions
   - vaccine

EXERCISE 1: FILL IN THE BLANK

Complete the following questions by writing the correct term(s) in the blank(s) provided.

1. The study of diseases that can cause abnormalities in the structure or function of various organ systems is

   _____.

2. The measurable characteristics the patient exhibits as a result of the disease process are referred to as

   _____.

3. The characteristics that the patient feels and describes as his/her condition as a result of a disease process are

   _____.

4. Alterations of cell growth are known as _____.

1

5. Adverse patient conditions caused by physicians and their treatment are known as _____.

6. Determining the precise disease process affecting the patient is known as _____.

7. In some cases the underlying cause is unknown, and this type of disease is termed _____.

8. Describing the expected patient outcomes is called _____.

9. Infections contracted at a healthcare facility are _____ infections.

10. Contagious diseases contracted outside the healthcare facility are known as _____.

11. The immediate response the body tissue has to a local injury is _____.

12. As a result of inflammation, there are four overlapping responses, which are:

    a. _____

    b. _____

    c. _____

    d. _____

13. The term _____ indicates the membrane has the ability to allow fluids to pass from one structure to another.

14. Inflammatory _____ causes the swelling associated with the inflammatory process, resulting in pressure and pain caused by protein-rich fluid.

15. Fibrous scar tissue replaces destroyed tissue with _____ tissue.

16. Fibrous scars are a result of strong connective tissue contracting to form a(n) _____ in the abdomen.

17. A protruding tumorlike scar, a(n) _____, results from an accumulation of excessive amounts of collagen.

18. List the five clinical signs of acute inflammation.

    a. _____

    b. _____

    c. _____

    d. _____

    e. _____

19. Microcirculation at the injury site results in _____ and _____.

20. Swelling occurs because the _____ increases the amount of interstitial fluid.

21. As a result of the swelling, the pressure on the nerve endings causes _____ and possible _____.

22. The presence of _____ bacteria leads to the production of pus containing dead white blood cells, inflammatory exudate, and bacteria.

23. The specific inflammation associated with pus formation is _____.

24. A(n) _____ is the result of encapsulation of a pyogenic infection.

25. When a pyogenic microorganism invades the blood vessel, _____ may cause involvement of other organs or tissues in the body.

26. An abnormal accumulation of fluid in intercellular tissue spaces or body cavities is known as _____.

27. The general accumulation of fluid throughout the body is _____.

28. Because of the effect of gravity, ambulatory patients tend to accumulate fluid in tissues around the _____ and _____.

29. Due to gravity, hospitalized patients who are nonambulatory or sedentary, fluid collects most prominently in their _____, _____, and _____.

30. An interference of the blood supply possibly caused by arterial narrowing or disease is _____.

31. Localized ischemic necrosis within a tissue or organ caused by poor vascular supply or drainage is caused by a(n) _____.

32. Thrombosis or embolic occlusions cause almost all _____.

33. The implication of a ruptured blood vessel is _____.

34. When a blood vessel ruptures and accumulates within body tissue, it results in a(n) _____.

35. A term that refers to the reduction of the size or number of cells in an organ or tissue is _____.

36. The failure of normal development accounting for a small size is _____ or _____.

37. When casted or immobilized, a limb may suffer a reduction of muscle mass, which is known as _____ atrophy.

38. _____, _____ atrophy may be caused by loss of innervation, by hormonal stimulation, or by decreased blood supply.

39. Hypertrophy indicates an increase in the size of cells, whereas an increase in the number of cells is referred to as _____.

40. A loss of uniformity of cells and their orientation, associated with prolonged irritation or inflammation, is _____.

41. "New growth" infused with abnormal proliferation of cells that are out of control is known as _____.

42. The study of neoplasms, also known as tumors, is _____.

43. Neoplastic growths closely resembling the cells of origin in structure and function are considered _____ tumors.

44. New growths invading and destroying adjacent structures that spread to distant sites are _____ neoplasms.

45. Malignant tumors are collectively known as _____.

46. Neoplasia consists of two basic components, which are the _____ and _____.

47. The name of a tumor is determined by the _____ tissue.

48. A benign tumor consisting of fibrous tissue is called a(n) _____.

49. Benign epithelial neoplasms with glandular characteristics are _____.

50. Malignant neoplasms of epithelial origin are called _____.

51. Adenocarcinoma refers to a malignancy of _____ tissue.

52. Malignant connective tissue neoplasms are_____, which tend to spread more rapidly than carcinomas.

53. Malignant neoplastic dissemination can occur by one of three pathways: _____, _____, and _____.

54. A tumor that penetrates the wall of the organ of origin and implants at distant sites is disseminated by _____.

55. _____ is assessing tumor aggressiveness (biologic behavior) or degree of malignancy, whereas _____ describes extensiveness of the tumor at the primary site and the presence or absence of metastases.

56. A study of determinants compiled for a specific disease in a given population determining the type of neoplastic involvement is _____.

57. The rate that an illness or abnormality occurs is _____.

58. Diseases that pass from one generation to the next through genetic information are known as _____ diseases.

59. _____ genes always produce a particular trait, and _____ genes manifest the particular trait when contributed by both parents.

60. When alterations occur in the DNA structure, _____ may result.

61. _____ react to foreign substances and bind to make antigens harmless.

62. Antibodies must have bound to antigens to develop _____.

63. _____ consist of dead or deactivated bacteria or viruses, whereas a(n) _____ is a chemically altered toxin.

64. An immune deficiency attributable to infection through retroviruses such as HIV is known as _____

_____ _____.

EXERCISE 2: MATCHING

Match each of the following terms with the correct definition by placing the letter of the best answer in the space provided. Each question has only one correct answer. Please note that there are more terms than definitions.

1. _____ disease caused by physician or treatment

2. _____ feelings that the patient describes— subjective manifestations

3. _____ infections contracted in a public setting outside of the acute care facility

4. _____ linked combination of signs and symptoms

5. _____ measurable or objective manifestations

6. _____ probable patient outcome

7. _____ study of the cause of the disease process

8. _____ underlying cause is unknown

A. asymptomatic

B. community-acquired infections

C. diagnosis

D. etiology

E. iatrogenic

F. idiopathic

G. nosocomial infections

H. prognosis

I. signs

J. symptoms

K. syndrome

Match each of the following terms with the correct definition by placing the letter of the best answer in the space provided. Each question has only one correct answer. Please note that there are more terms than definitions.

1. _____ assessing the aggressiveness of a malignant tumor

2. _____ consists of a low dose of dead or deactivated bacteria or viruses

3. _____ coughing up blood

4. _____ critical reaction that can cause death

5. _____ difficulty in swallowing

6. _____ epithelial tumor that grows as a projecting mass arising on the skin or on a mucous membrane

7. _____ foreign substances produced by invading organisms

8. _____ large, cystic, benign tumor masses

9. _____ loss of appetite

10. _____ major metastatic route of carcinomas

11. _____ malignant neoplasms of epithelial cell origin

12. _____ malignant tumors from connective tissue, such as bone, muscle, and cartilage

13. _____ opportunistic infection

14. _____ refers to extensiveness of a tumor and whether or not it has metastasized

15. _____ soft fatty tumors

16. _____ tumor cells grow well; patient becomes weak and emaciated

17. _____ tumors composed of blood vessels

18. _____ tumors of muscle

19. _____ use of cytotoxic substances that kill neoplastic cells and may cause injury to normal cells

20. _____ without form (cells)

A. anaphylactic

B. anaplastic

C. angiomas

D. anorexia

E. antigen

F. benign

G. cachexia

H. carcinomas

I. chemotherapy

J. cystadenomas

K. dysphagia

L. edema

M. grading

N. hematoma

O. hemoptysis

P. lipomas

Q. lymphatic

R. myomas

S. *Pneumocystis carinii* pneumonia

T. polyp

U. sarcomas

V. staging

W. vaccine

EXERCISE 4: MULTIPLE CHOICE

Circle the best answer for the following multiple choice questions.

1. The study of diseases that can cause abnormalities in the structure or function of various organ systems is
   a. oncology
   b. physiology
   c. pathology
   d. biology

2. A disease with an unknown cause is referred to as
   a. iatrogenic
   b. idiopathic
   c. nosocomial
   d. community acquired

3. A low-protein fluid that builds up in the tissue such as seen in pulmonary edema is
   a. hyperemia
   b. exudate
   c. transudate
   d. phagocytosis

4. The technologist may find it necessary to decrease technical factors to demonstrate which destructive disease?
   a. edema
   b. emphysema
   c. empyema
   d. exostosis

5. The type of microorganism that leads to the production of thick, yellow fluid called pus, which contains dead white blood cells, inflammatory exudate, and bacteria, is
   a. pyogenic bacteria
   b. a virus
   c. phagocytosis
   d. a fungus

6. A localized encapsulated collection of pus is called a(n)
   a. granuloma
   b. scar
   c. keloid
   d. abscess

7. An accumulation of abnormal amounts of fluid in the intercellular tissue spaces or body cavities is
   a. edema
   b. elephantiasis
   c. anasarca
   d. filariasis

8. A localized area of ischemic necrosis within a tissue or organ produced by occlusion of the arterial supply or venous drainage is
   a. a hematoma
   b. filariasis
   c. edema
   d. an infarct

9. A blood vessel rupture that is trapped within body tissue results in
   a. a hemorrhage
   b. a hematoma
   c. a hyperemia
   d. edema

10. What is indicated by an increase in the size of the cells in the tissue or organ in response to the body's demand for increased function?
    a. hyperplasia
    b. hypoplasia
    c. hypertrophy
    d. dysplasia

11. These make up the 44 chromosomes that contain thousands of genes, with the exception of the X or Y chromosome.
    a. homozygous genes
    b. autosomes
    c. heterozygous genes
    d. variable expressivity genes

12. Dominant genes _____ produce an effect regardless of their homozygous or heterozygous status.
    a. always
    b. frequently
    c. infrequently
    d. never

13. An alteration in the DNA structure, a(n) _____, can be caused by radiation, chemicals, or viruses.
    a. gene
    b. expression
    c. mutation
    d. autosome

14. Foreign substances such as bacteria, viruses, fungi, and toxins are called
    a. antibodies
    b. immunoglobulins
    c. antigens
    d. histamines

Chapter **1** **Introduction to Pathology**

15. Reviewing the population involved in statistically determining the expected outcome or death rate is called
    a. morbidity rate
    b. mortality rate
    c. epidemiology
    d. neoplastic staging

16. A systemic disease commonly resulting from AIDS that characteristically affects the skin is
    a. *Pneumocystis carinii* pneumonia
    b. Kaposi sarcoma
    c. hepatitis
    d. toxoplasmosis

SELF-TEST

Read each question carefully, then circle the best answer.

1. The body tissue's initial response to local injury is
   a. inflammation
   b. edema
   c. phagocytosis
   d. hemorrhage

2. The accumulation of abnormal amounts of fluid in the intercellular tissue is
   a. ischemia
   b. edema
   c. inflammation
   d. hemorrhage

3. Signs are
   a. what the patient feels
   b. characteristics that can be observed or measured
   c. the subjective symptoms the patient describes
   d. headaches and painful joints

4. The term used to describe the unknown cause of a disease process is
   a. iatrogenic
   b. community acquired
   c. nosocomial
   d. idiopathic

5. The interference of blood supply depriving organ cells and tissues of oxygen and nutrients is known as
   a. ischemia
   b. infarction
   c. anasarca
   d. filariasis

6. As a result of this process, a localized area of necrosis occurs within tissue or an organ, which is called
   a. ischemia
   b. infarction
   c. hemorrhage
   d. hypoplasia

7. What results in the accumulation of blood trapped within body tissue?
   a. hematoma
   b. hemorrhage
   c. infarction
   d. edema

8. An abnormal proliferation of cells outside the normal cell growth is known as
   a. cachexia
   b. cancer
   c. neoplasia
   d. sarcoma

9. If the genetic information contained in the nucleus of a cell causes abnormalities, it is considered
    a. an immunodeficiency disease
    b. an inflammatory disease
    c. a hereditary disease
    d. a neoplastic disease

10. Immunity can be attained by
    a. artificial means
    b. natural exposure
    c. vaccination
    d. all of the above

11. A disease process contracted in the healthcare facility is considered
    a. nosocomial
    b. idiopathic
    c. iatrogenic
    d. community acquired

12. Dysplasia is
    a. an increase in the size of cells
    b. an increase in the number of cells
    c. a loss of uniformity of individual cells
    d. a loss in the size and number of cells

13. There are four overlapping responses (blood flow, migration of white cells, digestion of dead cells and tissue, and repair) that cause
    a. edema
    b. inflammation
    c. hemorrhage
    d. infarction

14. Extravascular fluid in the lungs is known as
    a. pericardial effusion
    b. pulmonary effusion
    c. pulmonary edema
    d. hemothorax

15. An infarct can be caused by a thrombotic occlusion or a(n)
    a. hematoma
    b. hemorrhage
    c. granuloma
    d. embolism

16. Hemorrhage implies that a(n) _____ has occurred.
    a. interruption in the blood supply
    b. ischemic necrosis within tissue
    c. initial response to injury
    d. rupture of a blood vessel

17. In response to physiologic stimuli, cells may change in
    a. number
    b. size
    c. differentiation
    d. all of the above

18. Failure of cell development causes
    a. hyperplasia
    b. hypoplasia
    c. dysplasia
    d. neoplasia

Chapter **1** **Introduction to Pathology**

19. Neoplasms that invade and destroy adjacent structures and spread to distant sites are
    a. benign tumors
    b. malignant tumors
    c. metastatic tumors
    d. fatty tumors

20. Determining the extensiveness of a tumor at its primary site and the presence or absence of metastasis refers to
    a. staging
    b. grading
    c. hematogenous spread
    d. lymphatic spread

21. Hereditary disorders that may not affect parents and occur only when a person is homozygous for the defective gene are
    a. autosomal dominant disorders
    b. dominant disorders
    c. mutation disorders
    d. autosomal recessive disorders

22. A type of artificial immunity that exposes a person to dead or deactivated bacteria or viruses is
    a. active immunity
    b. passive immunity
    c. community-acquired immunity
    d. antigen immunity

23. PPE involves
    a. using the correct personal protective equipment
    b. minimizing exposure to healthcare workers
    c. following the Centers for Disease Control and Prevention's Standard Precautions
    d. utilizing all the information provided in answers a to c

24. Transmission-based diseases can be transmitted by
    a. contact
    b. droplet
    c. vector
    d. all of the above

25. HIV is the main cause of
    a. hepatitis C
    b. AIDS
    c. hepatitis A
    d. none of the above

2 Specialized Imaging Techniques

OBJECTIVES

In addition to the objectives listed at the beginning of Chapter 2 in the textbook, the user should be able to:

1. Describe briefly the theory of image production for the following specialties:
   - computed tomography (CT)
   - fusion imaging
   - magnetic resonance imaging (MRI)
   - mammography
   - nuclear medicine (NM)
   - positron emission tomography (PET)
   - single-photon emission computed tomography (SPECT)
   - ultrasound (US)

2. Classify the following terms as related to specific imaging modalities:
   - anechoic
   - angiography
   - annihilation
   - attenuation
   - biologic/molecular map
   - CT number
   - diffusion imaging
   - direct fusion
   - echo time (TE)
   - echogenic
   - full-field digital mammography (FFDM)
   - functional MRI
   - gamma camera
   - gamma ray
   - helical or spiral scan
   - high signal intensity
   - hyperechoic
   - hypoechoic
   - increased uptake
   - integrated imaging
   - isoechoic
   - low signal intensity
   - maximum intensity projections (MIPs)
   - multidetector scanning
   - physiologic map
   - positron
   - radiofrequency (RF)
   - radiopharmaceutical
   - repetition time (TR)
   - T1/T2-weighted image
   - tomography
   - virtual reality (VR)
   - volume-rendered imaging

EXERCISE 1: FILL IN THE BLANK

Complete the following questions by writing the correct term(s) in the blank(s) provided:

1. Common terminology that the radiologist uses to describe the image are the _____ _____.

2. The descriptor indicating the site where anatomic changes are evident is the _____.

3. The degree of vascularity of the abnormal tissues is described as the _____ of the tissue.

4. The most common imaging technique for diagnosing breast tissue today is _____ .

5. A noninvasive imaging modality, _____uses high-frequency sound waves produced by electrical stimulation of a specialized crystal.

6. _____ is the modality of choice for examinations of children and pregnant women in whom a potential danger exists from the radiation exposure involved with other imaging studies.

Chapter **2** **Specialized Imaging Techniques**

7. CT stands for _____ _____, which uses a computer to produce cross-sectional tomographic images of various soft tissues.

8. The first alternative to image the brain was provided by _____ _____, which eventually replaced pneumoencephalography.

9. Scientists integrated strong magnets and radiofrequencies to develop _____ _____ _____.

10. Researchers developed a positron-emitting radiopharmaceutical to produce molecular images to create _____, which stands for _____ _____ _____.

11. The modality that combines digital images using hybrid equipment or special software is _____ imaging.

12. Sound waves produced by a transducer describe the imaging theory of _____.

13. Sound waves passing through a water-tissue interface can produce reflections. These reflections are called _____.

14. In US, tissues transmitting sound waves easily are _____.

15. Strong reflections in US are called _____ or _____.

16. When two structures have the same echogenicity, the term _____ is used to describe them.

17. Doppler imaging is used to study _____ _____ _____ _____.

18. In Doppler imaging, color is used to represent the _____ of flow and _____.

19. Examples of acoustic barriers in US are _____ and _____.

20. Scanning using a narrow x-ray beam and computation of the attenuation coefficient, which is then displayed as a gray scale on the monitor, is _____.

21. The _____ reflects the specific tissue attenuation as relative to water in CT.

22. The highest CT number represents _____ and is _____.

23. The areas that appear black on CT have the _____ CT number, denoting _____.

24. High-resolution CT uses thin sections (_____ mm) to produce a very detailed display of lung anatomy.

25. Multiple single-scan CT equipment has been replaced by _____ or _____ scanners.

26. The sixth-generation CT scanners perform multiple slices consisting of multidetectors producing _____ to _____ slices per rotation.

27. The seventh-generation scanner collects data using a _____ beam and is a _____ multi-detector scanner.

28. Integrating all image data in CT by using software to produce 3D images is _____ imaging.

29. To enhance the CT image, _____ projections highlight the brightest pixels, improving the image.

30. To produce MR images, the technologist selects a pulse sequence that includes the RF pulse and its timing, which is usually represented by the _____ time and _____ time.

31. The most commonly used pulse sequence in MRI is referred to as _____.

32. Fat tissue, subacute hemorrhage, and highly proteinaceous material cause a high signal intensity that appears bright on _____ MR images.

33. On MRI T2-weighted images, _____, _____, _____, and fast-flowing blood generate no signal, so they appear very dark on most imaging sequences.

34. _____ produces images in multiple planes without the use of ionizing radiation and receives no signal from bone.

35. _____ imaging relies on fast scanning techniques and rapid gradient switching to image the random movement of water molecules within the brain or other organs.

36. To differentiate fat from contrast material to highlight vascular structures, _____ imaging is used.

37. _____ MR imaging visualizes blood transit time to help determine circulation in viable tissue.

38. Injecting a radionuclide and detecting the gamma radiation describe _____ imaging.

39. The dose of _____ is calculated on the basis of the specific half-life and decay rate.

40. The decay of the radionuclide is detected for imaging purposes by a _____ camera.

41. An increase in uptake on an NM scan that is directly proportional to the emission of gamma radiation is known as a _____ _____.

42. The modality that gathers the tomographic information in which a detector(s) rotates 180 to 360 degrees around the patient, acquiring multiple projections, is known as _____ _____ _____ _____.

43. SPECT imaging is useful in evaluating _____ disorders, infections, tumors, _____, and neurologic disorders, such as seizures and trauma.

44. The _____ for PET is different from that for NM and SPECT in that it decays by the emission of a _____.

45. The production of two high-energy photons in opposite directions is known as _____.

46. PET is especially useful for imaging in _____, _____, and neurology.

47. In fusion imaging, _____ imaging is accomplished with the use of software and _____ fusion imaging is a result of hybrid equipment.

Chapter **2** **Specialized Imaging Techniques**

EXERCISE 2: MATCHING

Match each of the following terms with the correct definition by placing the letter of the best answer in the space provided. Each question has only one correct answer. Please note that there are more terms than definitions.

1. _____ a drug that emits radiation

2. _____ ability to combine images from different modalities into one image

3. _____ allows for faster imaging and easy reformatting in the coronal and sagittal planes in CT

4. _____ produces images with high soft tissue resolution through the use of magnets and RFs

5. _____ capable of producing images of the fetus without the use of ionizing radiation

6. _____ compiles images to provide a 3D CT image, which is especially useful in visualizing the vascular system

7. _____ CT numbers represent this value

8. _____ equipment designed to integrate multimodality images

9. _____ produces high-resolution images of the vascular system without the need for IV contrast material

10. _____ has a gantry and x-ray tube, which rotate, producing cross-sectional images

11. _____ hot spots indicate an increase in uptake that is directly proportional to the emission of gamma radiation

12. _____ imaging especially useful in determining metastases in oncology patients to determine treatment

13. _____ in US, the term used when the organ tissues are very similar

14. _____ localizes the specific regions of neurologic function of the brain

15. _____ NM imaging with the addition of a rotating gamma camera

16. _____ on T1-weighted images, fat, subacute hemorrhage, and intravenous contrast material produce this signal

17. _____ the most common pulsing sequence(s) used in MRI today

18. _____ radiopharmaceuticals are detected with this device

19. _____ the time between the end of the last RF pulse and the point when the receiving coil listens for the signal

20. _____ the value given to the amount of attenuation in CT

A. annihilation
B. attenuation
C. computed tomography (CT)
D. CT number
E. direct fusion
F. echo time (TE)
G. echogenic
H. functional MR
I. fusion imaging
J. gamma camera
K. gamma ray
L. helical or spiral scan
M. high signal intensity
N. hypoechoic
O. integrated imaging
P. isoechoic
Q. magnetic resonance imaging (MRI)
R. MR angiography
S. nuclear medicine (NM)
T. positron emission tomography (PET)
U. radiopharmaceutical
V. repetition time
W. single-photon emission computed tomography (SPECT)
X. T1/T2-weighted image
Y. ultrasound (US)
Z. volume-rendered imaging

EXERCISE 3: MATCHING—IMAGING MODALITIES AND FEATURES

Match each of the following terms with the correct definition by placing the letter of the best answer in the space provided. Each question has only one correct answer. Please note that there are more terms than definitions.

1. _____ 3D rendering demonstrating the surface or selected structures

2. _____ comparison of echo intensities for adjacent tissue

3. _____ diameter or width and length (mm or cm)

4. _____ heterogeneous (septate) or homogeneous (fluids)

5. _____ high signals (bright) include fat, subacute hemorrhage, melanin, slow-flowing blood, and IV contrast

6. _____ increased uptake directly proportional to the emission of gamma radiation

7. _____ indistinctly marginated (infiltration into surrounding tissue)

8. _____ nodular (tumor or lymph nodes) or reticular (resembling a net)

9. _____ relative to surrounding tissue (hyperdense or hypodense; radiolucent or radiopaque)

10. _____ three planes of colored images to demonstrate the biochemistry of tissue (biologic map)

A. Computed tomography (CT)

B. Demarcation

C. Density

D. Location

E. Magnetic resonance imaging (MRI)

F. Mammography

G. Nuclear medicine/SPECT

H. Perfusion

I. Positron emission tomography (PET)

J. Shape

K. Size

L. Structure

M. Ultrasound

EXERCISE 4: MULTIPLE CHOICE

Circle the best answer for the following multiple choice questions.

1. Screening mammography images include
   a. AP and lateral projections
   b. craniocaudal and mediolateral oblique projections
   c. craniocaudal and mediolateral projections
   d. craniocaudal, mediolateral oblique, and mediolateral projections

2. Imaging in ultrasound relies on a(n)
   a. magnet and coil to send and receive radiofrequencies
   b. radioisotope to create an image
   c. transducer to receive and send sound waves
   d. x-ray and detectors to produce the image

3. Air and bone are _____ in ultrasound.
   a. hyperechoic
   b. anechoic
   c. acoustic barriers
   d. isoechoic

4. Helical scanning uses
   a. conventional single-slice scans
   b. table movement during scanning
   c. continuous x-ray exposure during scanning
   d. b and c

5. Cross-sectional images produced by high-frequency sound waves is the modality known as
   a. US
   b. CT
   c. MRI
   d. SPECT

6. In US, the transducer
   a. records the changes in signal pitch and direction
   b. is made of tungsten
   c. produces high-frequency sound waves
   d. a and c

Chapter **2** **Specialized Imaging Techniques**

7. Tissue that is echo free or lacking in signal is
   a. anechoic
   b. echogenic
   c. hyperechoic
   d. isoechoic

8. The CT number represents the
   a. attenuation of specific tissue relative to water
   b. signal intensity
   c. tissue echogenicity
   d. radionuclide concentration

9. The CT number representing bone (appearing white) is
   a. −1000
   b. 0
   c. 1250
   d. 1000

10. High-resolution CT
    a. requires a section thickness of 5 to 10 mm
    b. requires thin section slices of 1 mm
    c. decreases resolution
    d. increases volume artifact

11. In CT, the images that demonstrate the inside of a structure through reconstruction are called
    a. attenuation of specific tissue relative to water
    b. signal intensity
    c. virtual reality
    d. minimum intensity projections

12. The modality of choice for the spine and central nervous system is
    a. US
    b. CT
    c. MRI
    d. SPECT

13. The time it takes to play out the entire set of RF pulses before repeating is
    a. repetition time
    b. echo time
    c. RF pulsing
    d. a T1-weighted image

14. On MRI, blood flow generates
    a. no signal
    b. high signal intensity
    c. low signal intensity
    d. bright reflection

15. Tissue suppression in MRI
    a. creates a greater difference in tissue contrast
    b. is used in the neck, abdomen, and pelvis
    c. helps to differentiate tumor from normal tissue when the tissues are close in consistency
    d. all of the above

16. Molecular movement and random thermal motion are what _____ MR images rely on to produce an image.
    a. diffusion
    b. fat-suppressed
    c. functional
    d. spectroscopic

17. Gamma radiation detected by a gamma camera is emitted by
    a. gadolinium chelates
    b. iodinated contrast agents
    c. radiopharmaceuticals
    d. none of the above

18. In the gamma camera, when the gamma rays interact with the crystals, they produce
    a. electromagnetic frequencies
    b. light rays
    c. radiation
    d. sound waves

19. The advantage of NM is that
    a. a physiologic map is produced
    b. an anatomic map is produced
    c. earlier detection of a disease process is produced in comparison with plain radiographs
    d. all of the above

20. The major difference between SPECT and NM procedures is that
    a. NM produces a 3D image, whereas SPECT does not
    b. SPECT cameras rotate independently around the patient, whereas the NM gamma camera is stationary
    c. NM uses radiopharmaceuticals that produce higher doses than those used in SPECT
    d. There are no differences between NM scans and SPECT scans

21. In PET scanning, the radiopharmaceutical produces
    a. a neutron
    b. a positron
    c. an electron
    d. an x-ray

22. The modality that best demonstrates treatment results and is the most effective to illustrate recurring tumor growth is
    a. MRI
    b. SPECT
    c. NM
    d. PET

23. The modality that has been found to best demonstrate the physiologic changes in Alzheimer disease is
    a. MRI
    b. SPECT
    c. CT
    d. PET

24. The imaging modality that best demonstrates molecular-physiologic and anatomic relationships is
    a. fusion imaging
    b. PET
    c. CT
    d. SPECT

SELF-TEST

Read each question carefully, then circle the best answer.

1. The modality to best demonstrate the fetus without the use of ionizing radiation is
    a. CT
    b. MRI
    c. NM
    d. US

2. Computed tomography provides a
    a. cross-sectional view of anatomy
    b. physiologic map
    c. molecular map
    d. superimposed image of anatomic structures

3. The modality that provides three-dimensional images (axial, coronal, and sagittal) using RF pulses is
    a. US
    b. CT
    c. MRI
    d. NM

4. Using a radiopharmaceutical, computer, and rotating gamma camera provides diagnosticians with
    a. a cross-sectional view of anatomy
    b. a three-dimensional physiologic map
    c. anterior and posterior nuclear medicine images
    d. a three-dimensional anatomic map

5. The development of a radiopharmaceutical that emits positrons and the ability of gamma camera movement resulted in
    a. CT
    b. SPECT
    c. PET
    d. MRI

6. Echoes received by the transducer are the result of interaction between
    a. sounds and tissue
    b. RFs and a magnet
    c. x-ray and detectors
    d. radionuclides and a gamma camera

Chapter **2** **Specialized Imaging Techniques**

7. Tissue that produces a relatively strong reflection (echo) and appears as a bright intensity is said to be
   a. anechoic
   b. hyperechoic
   c. hypoechoic
   d. isoechoic

8. The best and safest mode to visualize blood flow, direction, and velocity is
   a. US
   b. SonoCT real-time compound imaging
   c. MRI
   d. Doppler imaging

9. Radiographic differentiation of soft tissue using a narrow collimated x-ray beam is accomplished by
   a. MRI
   b. CT
   c. SPECT
   d. PET

10. The ability to differentiate tissue in CT depends on the relative linear attenuation coefficient, which is referred to as
    a. the attenuation factor
    b. the calibration number
    c. the CT number
    d. echogenicity

11. CT scanning in a continuous mode using pitch variability
    a. depends on multidetectors
    b. depends on spiral or helical x-ray rotations and multidetectors
    c. indicates the use of conventional single-slice scanning protocols
    d. provides subsecond scanning abilities
    e. b and d

12. The most commonly used pulse sequences in MRI are termed
    a. echo time
    b. RF pulses
    c. repetition time
    d. spin-echo

13. The T1-weighted image depends on sequences with
    a. short TE and short TR pulses
    b. short TE and long TR pulses
    c. long TE and short TR pulses
    d. long TE and long TR pulses

14. On T2-weighted images, water appears
    a. as a high signal intensity
    b. as a low signal intensity
    c. as a dark region
    d. none of the above

15. MR angiography requires the use of
    a. a radionuclide to demonstrate the blood vessels
    b. administration of gadolinium contrast agent
    c. administration of an iodinated contrast agent
    d. administration of a microbubble contrast agent

16. Signals radiating from the patient are how _____ images are created.
    a. CT
    b. NM
    c. MRI
    d. US

17. Radionuclides
    a. emit high-frequency sound waves
    b. emit ionizing radiation
    c. produce complications similar to those caused by radiographic iodinated contrast agents
    d. have pharmacologic side effects

18. The sodium iodide crystals detect _____ to create an image.
    a. gamma rays
    b. high-frequency radio waves
    c. high-frequency sound waves
    d. x-rays

19. Diagnostic mammography imaging involves which of the following series of projections?
    a. full-field digital images
    b. craniocaudal, mediolateral oblique, and mediolateral images
    c. mediolateral oblique, and mediolateral images only
    d. craniocaudal and mediolateral images only

20. The gamma camera contains _____ crystals, which produce light.
    a. meglumine iodine
    b. selenium
    c. silver halide
    d. sodium iodide

21. Applying postprocessing in CT to amplify the brightest pixels produces a
    a. virtual reality image
    b. minimum intensity projection
    c. maximum intensity projection
    d. shaded surface-rendered image

22. In SPECT, the device that detects the radiation emitted from the patient is the
    a. gantry
    b. gamma camera
    c. receiving coil
    d. transducer

23. True or False. Computer-aided detection (CAD) can sometimes suggest abnormalities that are proven to not exist (false positives).

Chapter **2 Specialized Imaging Techniques**

24. AI can assist radiologists in calculating bone age for which type of pediatric examination?
   a. chest
   b. knees
   c. hands
   d. ankles

25. Which type of medical approach uses genetic testing to identify risk factors for certain conditions and employ targeted therapies for treatment?
   a. Alternative medicine
   b. Personalized medicine
   c. Perfusion imaging
   d. Diffusion imaging

3 Respiratory System

OBJECTIVES

In addition to the objectives listed at the beginning of Chapter 3 in the textbook, the user should be able to:
1. Identify anatomic structures on diagrams and radiographs of the respiratory system.
2. Describe the physiology of the respiratory system.
3. Differentiate the pathologic disorders of the respiratory system by defining the disease processes and their radiographic manifestations.
4. Determine changes in technical factors to obtain optimal-quality radiographs for patients with various underlying pathologic conditions.
5. Locate placement for an endotracheal tube, central venous catheter, Swan-Ganz catheter, and transvenous cardiac pacemaker.
6. Recognize the most common complications involved with improper placement of the aforementioned catheters and how chest radiography plays an important role in the diagnosis of these complications.

EXERCISE 1: LABELING—ANATOMY

Identify the anatomic structures indicated by writing the correct names in the spaces provided.

A. Structure plan of the respiratory system. The *inset* shows the alveolar sacs where the interchange of oxygen and carbon dioxide takes place through the walls of the grapelike alveoli.

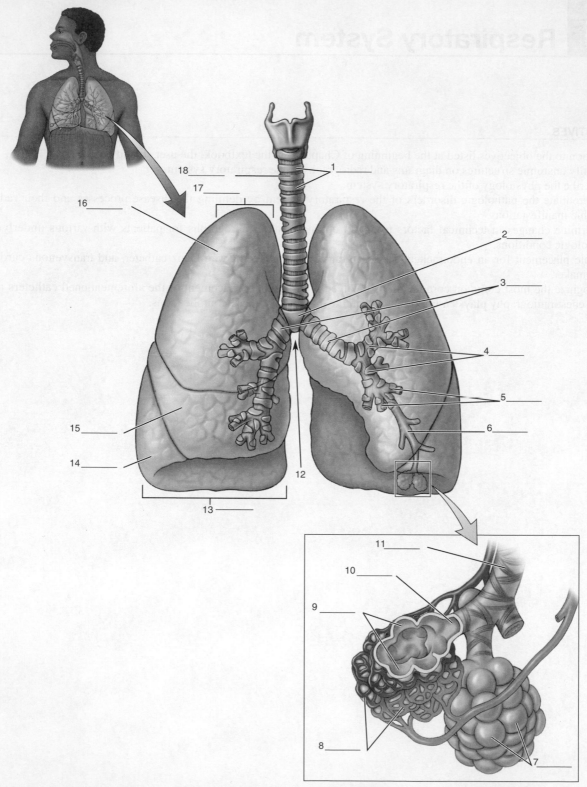

(From Herlihy B: *The human body in health and illness*, ed 6, St. Louis, 2018, Mosby.)

B. Lungs and pleura (transverse section). Note the parietal pleura lines the right and left pleural divisions of the thoracic cavity before folding inward near the bronchi to cover the lungs as the visceral pleura. The intrapleural space separates the parietal and visceral pleura. The heart, esophagus, and aorta are shown in the central mediastinum.

(From Thibodeau GA, Patton KT: *Anatomy and physiology*, ed 7, St. Louis, 2010, Mosby.)

EXERCISE 2: FILL IN THE BLANK—PHYSIOLOGY

Complete the following questions by writing the correct term(s) in the blank(s) provided.

1. The two major functions of the respiratory system are _____ and _____.

2. The lower respiratory system consists of _____, _____, and _____.

3. The lower respiratory system is responsible for _____ from the upper respiratory system.

4. The tracheobronchial tree is lined with a _____ _____.

5. The tracheobronchial tree contains _____ projections called cilia.

6. _____ prevent dust and foreign particles from reaching the lungs.

7. When cilia permit particles to enter the respiratory system (because of damage), the particles _____ to produce a disease process.

8. External respiration occurs in the _____.

9. Oxygen attaches to the _____ molecules in the red blood cells to circulate to various tissues throughout the body; this process is considered _____ respiration.

10. The _____ and _____ muscles are stimulated to contract, causing the lungs to _____.

11. Pulmonary circulation provides the _____ with oxygenated blood.

12. The inner lining surrounding and attached to the lung wall is the _____ _____.

EXERCISE 3: FILL IN THE BLANK—RESPIRATORY PATHOLOGY

Complete the following questions by writing the correct term(s) in the blank(s) provided.

1. Irregular thickening of linear chest markings due to excessively viscous mucus is the radiographic appearance in

   _____ _____.

2. _____ consists of lipoproteins and provides the proper surface tension in the alveoli, allowing full external respirations.

3. On lateral projections of the neck using soft tissue techniques, a rounded thickening of the epiglottic shadow gives

   it the configuration and approximate size of an adult's thumb in the radiographic appearance of _____ disorder.

4. _____ is characterized by the cause and location of the disease process in the lung.

5. A lung abscess appears as a _____ density characteristically having a _____

   _____ periphery.

6. A bacterium that is rod-shaped with a waxy coat allowing it to live outside the body for an extended time is

   _____ _____.

7. Pulmonary infiltration(s), most commonly in the periphery of the parenchyma, which may resemble pneumonia, are

   the radiographic appearance of _____.

8. _____ is estimated to affect almost all children by age 2 years and appears on chest radiographs as hyperinflation with diffuse increased interstitial markings.

9. Emphysema, chronic bronchitis, and asthma are examples of _____ _____.

10. Bilateral, symmetrical hilar lymph node enlargement is the classic radiographic abnormality in _____.

11. In _____, the lung reacts to occupational exposure to silica, which results in extensive fibrosis.

12. _____ causes peripheral atelectasis and pneumonitis as a result of bronchial obstruction.

13. An abnormal vascular communication between the pulmonary artery and the pulmonary vein is a pulmonary

    _____ _____.

EXERCISE 4: MATCHING—ANATOMY AND PHYSIOLOGY

Match each of the following terms with the correct definition by placing the letter of the best answer in the space provided. Each question has only one correct answer. Please note that there are more terms than definitions.

1. _____ breathing that supplies oxygen-rich air to the alveoli

2. _____ carbon dioxide regulates the respiration center in the brain

3. _____ cluster of alveoli

4. _____ consists of nasopharynx, oropharynx, and larynx

5. _____ extremely thin-walled sacs surrounded by blood capillaries

6. _____ fluid in the pleural space

7. _____ membrane attached to the inner chest wall (thoracic cavity)

8. _____ oxygen and carbon dioxide exchange caused as a result of cellular metabolism

9. _____ oxygenates blood and removes body waste such as carbon dioxide

10. _____ prevents dust and foreign particles from reaching the lungs

11. _____ provides the lung tissue with oxygen and nourishment

12. _____ respiratory muscles relaxing cause the lungs to expel air

A. acinus

B. bronchial circulation

C. cilia

D. expiration

E. external respiration

F. inspiration

G. internal respiration

H. lower respiratory system

I. medulla

J. mucous membrane

K. parenchyma

L. parietal pleura

M. pleural effusion

N. pulmonary circulation

O. pulmonary edema

P. upper respiratory system

Q. visceral pleura

Match each of the following terms with the correct definition by placing the letter of the best answer in the space provided. Each question has only one correct answer. Please note that there are more terms than definitions.

1. _____ abnormal communication between the pulmonary arteries and veins

2. _____ air bronchogram is the radiographic appearance because of immature lung development

3. _____ arises from thrombi in the deep venous system

4. _____ condition of a collapsed lung

5. _____ consolidation of the lung parenchyma sometimes causing an air bronchogram

6. _____ diseases caused by prolonged occupational exposure to irritating particulates causing interstitial inflammation

7. _____ fungal infection of the lung

8. _____ hereditary disease noted for secreting excessive viscous mucus by all endocrine glands

9. _____ most common type of lung cancer, typically arising in the major bronchi

10. _____ multisystem granulomatous disease

11. _____ necrotic area of pulmonary parenchyma containing purulent material

12. _____ neoplastic growth that is the result of an inflammatory process

13. _____ permanent irreversible obstructive and destructive changes in the acini

14. _____ primary carcinoma originating in the mucosa of the bronchial tree

15. _____ pus in the pleural cavity

16. _____ several conditions in which chronic obstruction of the airways leads to ineffective external respiration

17. _____ thin fibers embed in the lung, causing major fibrosis; may result in mesothelioma

18. _____ a disease that has four primary radiographic appearances: infiltrates, hilar enlargement, Ghon lesions, and pleural effusion

19. _____ viral inflammatory obstruction of the subglottic area of the trachea

20. _____ virus causing necrosis of the respiratory epithelium in the lower respiratory system

21. _____ widespread narrowing of airways caused by an increased response of the tracheobronchial tree to various allergens

A. asbestosis

B. asthma

C. atelectasis

D. benign granuloma

E. bronchial adenoma

F. bronchogenic carcinoma

G. chronic obstructive pulmonary disease

H. croup

I. cystic fibrosis

J. emphysema

K. empyema

L. hyaline membrane disease

M. lung abscess

N. pneumoconiosis

O. pneumonia

P. pulmonary arteriovenous fistula

Q. pulmonary emboli

R. pulmonary mycosis

S. respiratory syncytial virus

T. sarcoidosis

U. squamous carcinoma

V. tuberculosis

EXERCISE 6: MULTIPLE CHOICE

Circle the best answer for each of the following multiple choice questions.

1. Placement of the endotracheal tube should be evident on a radiograph at
   a. the carina
   b. 3 to 5 cm above the carina
   c. 10 to 15 cm above the carina
   d. the mainstem bronchi

2. The ideal positions for the tip of a peripherally inserted central catheter (PICC) in the patient are
   a. left main pulmonary artery
   b. within the distal superior vena cava
   c. above the cavoatrial junction
   d. b and c

3. To best demonstrate possible air-fluid levels in a lung abscess, the technologist should perform chest images with the patient
   a. upright
   b. semi-upright
   c. recumbent
   d. supine

4. Croup and epiglottitis are best demonstrated on
   a. AP and lateral neck images
   b. soft tissue AP and lateral neck images
   c. increased kV AP and lateral neck images
   d. Posteroanterior (PA) and lateral upright chest images

5. Consolidation of the lung parenchyma most commonly due to a virus or mycoplasma is
   a. bronchopneumonia
   b. interstitial pneumonia
   c. alveolar pneumonia
   d. tuberculosis

6. Pulmonary mycosis is caused by a
   a. virus
   b. bacterium
   c. fungus
   d. parasite

7. Respiratory epithelial necrosis leading to bronchiolitis and resulting in interstitial pneumonia is
   a. alveolar pneumonia
   b. RSV
   c. tuberculosis
   d. bronchial emphysema

8. Large bullae develop in end stage emphysema, causing a reduction of the lung parenchyma due to alveolar destruction, which requires the technologist to
   a. increase technical factors
   b. use routine technical factors
   c. increase exposure time
   d. decrease technical factors

9. Extended occupational exposure to small particulates that embed in the lung parenchyma is
   a. pneumoconiosis
   b. pulmonary mycosis
   c. chronic obstructive pulmonary disease
   d. tuberculosis

10. Pulmonary metastases that typically appear as multiple round or oval nodules throughout the lungs is a
    a. miliary type
    b. hematogenous type
    c. bronchial adenoma
    d. granuloma

11. The modality that helps determine whether a solitary nodule is benign is
    a. SPECT scan demonstrating a single hot spot
    b. PET scan detecting a single nodule with low cellular activity
    c. NM lung scan with decreased uptake in multiple lung segments
    d. CT scan demonstrating an irregular spiculated lesion

12. CT demonstrates pulmonary emboli as a(n)
    a. filling defect
    b. contrast-enhanced region
    c. area of abnormal increased blood flow
    d. irregular nodule

13. Bilateral symmetrical hilar lymph node enlargement is the classic radiographic appearance of
    a. systemic lupus erythematosus
    b. lead poisoning
    c. melanoma
    d. sarcoidosis

The problems described in the following case studies required imaging related to placement of an internal device. After each scenario, the images are presented and you will be asked to answer questions. Using your knowledge of imaging pathology and internal devices, apply exposure factors and positioning criteria to answer the questions.

CASE STUDY 1

A 45-year-old man underwent clinical follow-up imaging in the intensive care unit, which included a portable chest radiograph to evaluate his tracheostomy tube placement. See the following portable chest radiograph:

1. The purpose of the image is to locate the tracheostomy tube. Where is the tip of the tracheostomy tube?

2. The chest radiograph was taken with the patient in the recumbent position. Is this a concern when evaluating tube placement?

3. Because the radiograph was obtained with the patient in the recumbent position, what pathology could be missed?

4. In the mobile setting, if air-fluid levels need to be demonstrated, what positioning criteria are needed?

5. What is the other tube in the right lung called?

6. What is this other tube for?

CASE STUDY 2

A 40-year-old woman underwent clinical follow-up imaging in the intensive care unit, which included a portable chest radiograph, to evaluate placement of a Swan-Ganz catheter and a tracheostomy tube. See the following portable chest radiograph:

1. In this case, the external portion of the Swan-Ganz catheter is seen on the left shoulder. Can you identify the distal or internal placement of this catheter?

2. How would a radiographer viewing the radiograph determine whether the proper exposure factors have been used?

Chapter **3 Respiratory System**

3. One purpose of the image is to locate the tracheostomy tube. Where is the tip of the tube demonstrated?

4. If you look closely, you can see a tube in the patient's midline from the neck through the inferior chest (below the diaphragm). Because this tube appears to continue into the abdominal structures, what might the tube be?

Could this tube be the oxygen tubing?

5. What are the three lines that are crossing off to the left of the patient called?

Have these lines been moved sufficiently? Can the technologist disconnect these lines?

CASE STUDY 3

A 55-year-old man was experiencing shortness of breath (SOB), so a clinical follow-up radiograph was obtained. The patient previously had a coronary artery bypass graft (CABG). The following chest radiograph was obtained with the patient upright and on inspiration:

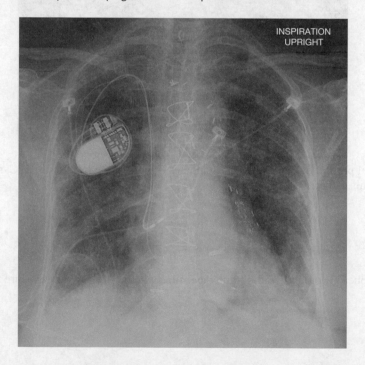

1. The pulse generator (pacemaker) can be seen in the right lung/shoulder region. Can you identify the distal or internal placement of the leads?

2. Are the electrocardiogram (EKG) leads interfering with identification of the pacer leads?

3. The most superior pacemaker lead would be located where?

4. The inferior pacemaker lead is located where?

CASE STUDY 4

An adult male patient entered the healthcare facility with dyspnea. The following chest radiograph was produced:

1. Was the chest radiograph completed in the upright position as per routine chest protocol?

2. How is it determined whether the chest radiograph was completed in the upright position?

3. Describe any subtle abnormalities seen.

4. Does the abnormality demonstrate air-fluid levels? If not, how would you describe it?

5. Were appropriate exposure factors used to demonstrate this pathologic condition?

6. Diagnosis is beyond the scope of radiographers' practice; however, the radiographer should be able to recognize that the image demonstrates abnormalities. Do you have any idea what disease process is being demonstrated here?

An 8-year-old boy entered the emergency department with a fever. The following PA and lateral chest radiographs were obtained:

Images were exposed using normal technical factors. The radiologist's interpretation denotes mild infiltrates in the left lower lobe. Clinical correlation was recommended. The patient was given antibiotic treatment.

Seventeen days later, the boy returned to the emergency department with difficulty breathing. More upright PA and lateral chest radiographs were completed, as follows:

1. In the current chest image, are there differences from the initial image? How would you describe what is shown?

2. What positioning criteria must be followed to demonstrate a true mediastinal shift? Why?

3. How does the image demonstrate upright positioning and the use of a horizontal beam?

4. What other images could be completed that would demonstrate fluid movement? In this case, what position would be most beneficial?

5. Diagnosis is beyond the scope of radiographers' practice; however, you should be able to recognize that the image demonstrates abnormalities. Do you have any idea what disease process is being demonstrated?

SELF-TEST

Read each question carefully, then circle the best answer.

1. The major function of the respiratory system is to
   (1) provide oxygen for the blood
   (2) remove oxygen from the body tissue
   (3) provide carbon dioxide to body tissue
   (4) remove carbon dioxide from the blood
      a. 1 and 2
      b. 1 and 4
      c. 2 and 3
      d. 3 and 4

2. The lower respiratory system consists of the
   a. nasopharynx
   b. trachea
   c. oropharynx
   d. larynx

34

3. The gas exchange in the lung takes place in the
   a. bronchi
   b. bronchioles
   c. capillaries
   d. alveoli

4. On full inspiration, the diaphragm projects at the level of the
   a. 6th anterior intercostal space
   b. 8th posterior intercostal space
   c. 10th anterior intercostal space
   d. 10th posterior intercostal space

5. A device that can measure the pulmonary capillary wedge pressure, cardiac output, and central venous pressure is a
   a. Swan-Ganz catheter
   b. CVP catheter
   c. peripherally inserted central catheter (PICC) line
   d. transvenous cardiac pacer

6. The disease process that is characterized by the secretion of excessive viscous mucus is
   a. cystic fibrosis
   b. tuberculosis
   c. hyaline membrane disease
   d. croup

7. Lack of lung development in premature infants that is radiographically demonstrated as an air bronchogram is
   a. cystic fibrosis
   b. tuberculosis
   c. hyaline membrane disease
   d. croup

8. Major radiographic signs are pulmonary overinflation, alterations in pulmonary vascularization, and bullae formation in
   a. chronic obstructive pulmonary disease
   b. emphysema
   c. asthma
   d. histoplasmosis

9. The most common work-related lung disease is
   a. silicosis
   b. anthracosis
   c. asbestosis
   d. pulmonary mycosis

10. Pneumoconiosis demonstrates radiographically as
    a. pleural effusion
    b. pulmonary edema
    c. scattered nodules and pleural thickening
    d. hemothorax

11. The severity of the pneumoconiosis depends on the
    a. size of the particles
    b. length of exposure
    c. concentration of particulates in the atmosphere
    d. a, b, and c are correct

12. Lung cancers originating in the glandular structures of the bronchial tree are known as
    a. bronchiolar carcinoma
    b. alveolar cell carcinoma
    c. bronchial adenoma
    d. bronchogenic carcinoma

13. A staphylococcal infection primarily in the bronchi or bronchiolar mucosa describes
    a. bronchopneumonia
    b. interstitial pneumonia
    c. aspiration pneumonia
    d. pulmonary mycosis

14. Pneumonia appears radiographically as a(n)
    a. opacification
    b. radiolucency
    c. decreased attenuated region
    d. encapsulated area with an air-fluid level

15. Tuberculosis survives outside the host for a long time because of its
    a. shape
    b. waxy coat
    c. size
    d. droplet spread

16. A disease of the lung caused by a fungus is
    a. pulmonary mycosis
    b. pneumoconiosis
    c. respiratory syncytial virus
    d. chronic obstructive pulmonary disease

17. As a result of epithelial necrosis, the radiograph demonstrates an interstitial pneumonia in cases of
    a. respiratory syncytial virus
    b. chronic obstructive pulmonary disease
    c. pulmonary mycosis
    d. pneumoconiosis

18. If an upright image cannot be obtained, what other position or view would demonstrate pleural effusion?
    a. cross-table lateral
    b. lateral decubitus
    c. transthoracic
    d. Trendelenburg

19. Which of the following chest pathologies requires a decrease in technical factors from a "normal" chest radiograph?
    a. atelectasis
    b. pleural effusion
    c. pneumonia
    d. pneumothorax

20. Which of the following chest pathologies requires an increase in technical factors from those used for a "normal" chest radiograph?
    a. atelectasis
    b. pulmonary edema
    c. pneumonia
    d. pneumothorax

21. Which of the following respiratory pathologies is not associated with chronic obstructive pulmonary disease?
    a. asthma
    b. bronchitis
    c. emphysema
    d. croup

22. Croup is
    a. a viral infection of the subglottis
    b. a thickened epiglottis
    c. a rounded thickening of the epiglottic shadow
    d. demonstrated best on a lateral soft tissue image

23. High-resolution CT has replaced V/Q scans in diagnosing
    a. pulmonary edema
    b. pulmonary effusion
    c. pulmonary emboli
    d. pulmonary mycosis

24. A filling defect seen in the pulmonary artery is indicative of
    a. pulmonary edema
    b. pulmonary effusion
    c. pulmonary emboli
    d. pulmonary mycosis

25. The abnormal connection between the pulmonary arteries and veins results in a pulmonary
    a. arteriovenous fistula
    b. effusion
    c. hemothorax
    d. embolism

26. The condition in which the lung collapses, causing reduced lung volume, is described as
    a. atelectasis
    b. pneumothorax
    c. hemothorax
    d. emphysema

27. Pneumothorax radiographically appears as
    a. an area without pulmonary markings
    b. fluid-filled pleura
    c. an air-fluid level in the lung parenchyma
    d. an enlarged heart

28. Thickened infected liquid or pus in the pleural space describes
    a. pleural effusion
    b. pleural edema
    c. empyema
    d. atelectasis

29. The mediastinum contains the following organs or structures:
    a. heart, great vessels, trachea, and thyroid gland
    b. heart, trachea, esophagus, and thyroid gland
    c. heart, mainstem bronchi, esophagus, and thymus gland
    d. heart, trachea, esophagus, and thymus gland

30. To best demonstrate the mediastinum, the chest image must be completed with
    a. no rotation, true PA positioning
    b. scapulae removed from the lung field
    c. AP positioning because the mediastinal structures are located anteriorly
    d. none of the above

31. Paradoxical movement of the diaphragm best demonstrated on fluoroscopy describes
    a. eventration of the diaphragm
    b. elevation of the diaphragm
    c. paralysis of the diaphragm
    d. normal movement of the diaphragm

4 Skeletal System

OBJECTIVES

In addition to the objectives listed at the beginning of Chapter 4 in the textbook, the user should be able to:
1. Identify anatomic structures on diagrams and radiographs of the skeletal system.
2. Describe the physiology of the skeletal system.
3. Differentiate the pathologic disorders of the skeletal system by defining the disease processes and their radiographic manifestations.
4. Determine changes in technical factors to obtain optimal-quality radiographs for patients with various underlying pathologic conditions.

EXERCISE 1: LABELING—ANATOMY

Identify the anatomic structures indicated by writing the correct names in the spaces provided.

A, Long bone.

(From Herlihy B: *The human body in health and illness*, ed 6, St. Louis, 2018, Mosby.)

B, Bone fracture and repair.

Fracture hematoma

1 _____

2 _____

A

B

3 _____

4 _____

(From Thibodeau GA, Patton KT: *Anatomy and physiology*, ed 6, St. Louis, 2007, Mosby.)

Name the stages of trauma as related to the previous figure.

1. Initial stage: _____

2. Results in _____

3. New bone formation: _____

4. Last stage: _____

EXERCISE 2: FILL IN THE BLANK—PHYSIOLOGY

Complete the following questions by writing the correct term(s) in the blank(s) provided.

1. The two highly specialized connective tissues in the skeletal system are _____ and _____.

2. The two major types of bone are _____ and _____.

3. The two membranes associated with bone are _____ and _____.

4. The compact bone appears _____ and _____.

5. Weblike bone structure consisting of marrow-filled spaces is _____ or _____ bone.

6. Cancellous bone appears as _____ on the radiographic image.

7. Linear bone growth occurs at the _____ plate.

8. The two special types of bone cells are _____ and _____.

9. The term for bone formation is _____, and the term for bone destruction is _____.

10. The skull and flat bones do not have a cartilaginous stage in bone formation; therefore, bone development occurs through _____ _____.

11. The diameter of the long bone expands or grows by _____ in the periosteum, producing new bone.

12. What five basic functions do bones perform?

    (i) _____

    (ii) _____

    (iii) _____

    (iv) _____

    (v) _____

EXERCISE 3: FILL IN THE BLANK—SKELETAL PATHOLOGY

Complete the following questions by writing the correct term(s) in the blank(s) provided.

1. A vertebra that has characteristics of the spinal column above and below is considered a _____ vertebra.

2. A splitting of the bony neural canal is referred to as _____.

3. The most common form of dwarfism is _____, which is the result of diminished proliferation of cartilage in the growth plate.

4. When the spine curves in a lateral direction, it is known as _____.

5. _____ is characterized pathologically by loss of joint cartilage and reactive new bone formation.

6. _____ is inflammation of the small fluid-filled sac located near the joint, the purpose of which is to reduce friction caused by movement.

7. A deep soft tissue swelling with obliteration or displacement of the fat planes and subtle metaphyseal lucencies describes _____.

8. Vitamin D deficiency in adults causes a loss of _____ as a result of the lack of calcium and phosphorus.

9. The chronic form of _____ may cause mental retardation, seizures, or delayed development.

10. The most common metabolic disease of the skeletal system is _____ disease, which affects both osteoblasts and osteoclasts.

11. A(n) _____ bone cyst contains numerous blood-filled arteriovenous communications.

12. The continuous external bridge of calcium deposit that extends across a fracture line is _____.

13. A fracture that may heal in a faulty position, resulting in impairment of function, is called _____.

14. _____ _____ is a chronic systemic disease of unknown cause, usually occurring in the small joints of the hands and feet.

EXERCISE 4: MATCHING—ANATOMY AND PHYSIOLOGY

Match each of the following terms with the correct definition by placing the letter of the best answer in the space provided. Each question has only one correct answer. Please note that there are more terms than definitions.

1. _____ bone formation from cartilage

2. _____ connective tissue bone formation

3. _____ dense structureless outer bone

4. _____ end of the shaft where the bone flares and becomes the epiphysis

5. _____ ends of long bones where growth occurs

6. _____ fibrous membrane covering the outer surface of bone

7. _____ ossification of flat bones on their outer surfaces

8. _____ membrane that lines the medullary cavity

9. _____ portion of bone where blood production occurs

10. _____ resorbing bone cells that enlarge the diameter of the medullary cavity

11. _____ shaftlike portion of bone

12. _____ area that contains trabeculae

A. appositional growth

B. compact bone

C. diaphysis

D. endosteum

E. epiphyseal cartilage

F. epiphysis

G. intramembranous ossification

H. medullary cavity

I. metaphysis

J. ossification

K. osteoblasts

L. osteoclasts

M. periosteum

N. resorption

O. spongy bone

P. trabeculae

EXERCISE 5: MATCHING—SKELETAL PATHOLOGY

Match each of the following terms with the correct definition by placing the letter of the best answer in the space provided. Each question has only one correct answer. Please note that there are more terms than definitions.

1. _____ cotton-wool skull appearance

2. _____ a cleft in the pars interarticularis between the superior and inferior articular processes in the vertebra

3. _____ a deposit of uric acid in the joint

4. _____ a malignant tumor of cartilaginous origin that may originate anew or within a preexisting cartilaginous lesion

5. _____ abnormal decrease in bone density due to lack of calcium deposits

6. _____ arises in the bone marrow of long bones and affects young adults

7. _____ benign bone projection with a cartilaginous cap

8. _____ brittle bone disease

9. _____ caused by vitamin deficiency in children

10. _____ classic "sunburst" pattern with elevated periosteum

11. _____ concentration deposited in the rapidly growing portions of bones, especially the metaphysis

12. _____ degenerative arthritis

13. _____ failure of cartilage to form properly, resulting in dwarfism

14. _____ infection of the bone and its marrow

15. _____ inflammation of the fluid-filled sac usually due to repeated physical activity

16. _____ lack of neural tube closure

17. _____ marble bone disease

18. _____ most commonly affects the thoracic and lumbar spine with poorly marginated bone destruction often associated with an abscess

19. _____ proliferation of fibrous tissue in the medullary cavity

20. _____ rupture of central nucleus pulposus, most frequently L4-L5

21. _____ true fluid-filled area surrounded by a fibrous wall

A. achondroplasia

B. bursitis

C. chondrosarcoma

D. Ewing sarcoma

E. fibrous dysplasia

F. gout

G. herniated intervertebral disk

H. hip dysplasia

I. lead poisoning

J. osteoarthritis

K. osteochondroma

L. osteogenesis imperfecta

M. osteogenic sarcoma

N. osteomalacia

O. osteomyelitis

P. osteopetrosis

Q. osteoporosis

R. Paget disease

S. Pott disease

T. rheumatoid arthritis

U. rickets

V. spina bifida

W. spondylolisthesis

X. spondylolysis

Y. unicameral bone cyst

Z. vertebral anomaly

EXERCISE 6: MATCHING—FRACTURE TERMS

Match each of the following terms with the correct definition by placing the letter of the best answer in the space provided. Each question has only one correct answer. Please note that there are more terms than definitions.

1. _____ bone response to repeated stresses

2. _____ composed of more than two fragments

3. _____ discontinuity between two or more fragments

4. _____ disruption of overlying skin

5. _____ encircles the bone shaft

6. _____ fracture healing process stops

7. _____ fragment torn from bony prominence

8. _____ incomplete fracture with the opposing cortex intact

9. _____ occurs at a right angle to the long axis of bone

10. _____ overlying skin is intact

11. _____ runs approximately 45 degrees to the bone shaft

12. _____ separation of bone fragments

A. avulsion

B. closed

C. comminuted

D. complete

E. displaced

F. fatigue

G. greenstick

H. malunion

I. nonunion

J. oblique

K. open

L. segmental

M. spiral

N. transverse

EXERCISE 7: MATCHING—TYPES OF FRACTURES

Match each of the following fractures with the correct definition by placing the letter of the best answer in the space provided. Each question has only one correct answer. Please note that there are more terms than definitions.

1. _____ ankle dislocation with fractured malleoli

2. _____ avulsion fracture at the base of the fifth metatarsal

3. _____ avulsion fracture of the spinous process

4. _____ C2 fracture of the arch, usually associated with anterior subluxation of C2-C3

5. _____ comminuted fracture of the ring of the atlas

6. _____ isolated fracture of the ulna with associated dislocation of the radius in the elbow

7. _____ transverse fracture of the lumbar vertebra

8. _____ transverse fracture of the neck of the fifth metacarpal

9. _____ transverse fracture of the waist of this carpal bone

10. _____ transverse fracture through the distal radius with dorsal angulation

A. boxer's

B. clay shoveler's

C. Colles

D. hangman's

E. Jefferson

F. Jones

G. Monteggia

H. navicular

I. Pott

J. seat belt

K. stress

L. torus

EXERCISE 8: MULTIPLE CHOICE

Circle the best answer for each of the following multiple choice questions.

1. The excessive proliferation of fibrous tissue in the medullary cavity describes
   a. achondroplasia
   b. fibrous dysplasia
   c. osteomalacia
   d. gout

2. The displacement of L4-L5 due to slippage of the inferior and superior intervertebral facets is
   a. spondylolysis
   b. spondylolisthesis
   c. a ruptured intervertebral disk
   d. a Jefferson fracture

3. A herniation of the meninges is
   a. a myelomeningocele
   b. a meningocele
   c. spina bifida occulta
   d. a Chiari II malformation

4. Bone that fails to resorb and causes a loss of bone marrow is referred to as
   a. osteomalacia
   b. osteoporosis
   c. osteopetrosis
   d. osteogenesis imperfecta

5. Severe osteoporosis and thin defective cortices resulting in multiple fractures occur in patients with
   a. osteomalacia
   b. osteoporosis
   c. osteopetrosis
   d. osteogenesis imperfecta

6. The hip may "pop" out of joint and a "click" may be felt or heard on clinical evaluation in children with
   a. chondromas
   b. herniated vertebral disks
   c. club feet
   d. congenital hip dysplasia

7. _____ may undergo spontaneous remission and has symmetrical involvement.
   a. Osteoarthritis
   b. Rheumatoid arthritis
   c. Psoriatic arthritis
   d. Infectious arthritis

8. In _____, localized bone deficiency occurs as a result of decreased bone mass per unit volume.
   a. osteoporosis
   b. osteomalacia
   c. osteopetrosis
   d. osteomyelitis

9. After repeated attacks, the inflammatory reaction produces evidence of joint effusion and clumps of crystal urate in patients affected with
   a. gout
   b. osteoarthritis
   c. pyogenic arthritis
   d. osteomyelitis

10. The disease process that results in the decreased absorption of calcium due to a vitamin deficiency is
    a. osteopetrosis
    b. osteomyelitis
    c. rickets
    d. scurvy

11. Osteochondromas are
    a. dense round lesions usually in the outer skull table
    b. growths parallel to the long axis of a bone
    c. usually found in the small bones of the hands and feet
    d. tumors that originate from osteoblastic cells in the bony cortices

12. Scoliosis is
    a. superoanterior vertebral displacement
    b. inferoposterior vertebral displacement
    c. lateral vertebral displacement
    d. posterior sacral displacement

13. Grade 1 spondylolisthesis as seen on the lateral projection refers to
    a. sacrum is displaced forward
    b. upper vertebral body displaced up to one-fourth the thickness of the lower vertebral body
    c. sacrum is displaced completely posteriorly from the fifth lumbar vertebra
    d. fifth lumbar vertebra is displaced anteriorly three quarters of the thickness of the sacrum

14. In the diagnosis of spondylolysis, which additional projections will be most helpful?
    a. standing AP and lateral lumbar spine projections
    b. oblique lumbar spine projections
    c. flexion and extension lateral lumbar spine projections
    d. standing flexion and extension lateral lumbar spine projections

The following case studies required skeletal imaging. After each scenario, the image(s) are presented and you will be asked to answer questions. Using the knowledge of imaging pathology, apply exposure factors and positioning criteria to answer the posed questions.

CASE STUDY 1

A patient enters the radiology department with an order for bilateral hand images. The patient has stiff and painful joints. Anteroposterior (AP) bilateral hand images were taken.

1. The interphalangeal joints should appear open on posteroanterior (PA) hand images. Name two positioning criteria to accomplish opening these joints.

2. When the patient cannot place palmar surface of the hands flat on the image receptor for a routine PA projection, what alternate projection(s) might better open the interphalangeal joints?

3. The joints appear to be enlarged as a result of effusion and to be misaligned. Name the category that this disease process is associated with.

4. What is the differential diagnosis?

A young patient enters the radiography department with an order for bilateral lower leg images. The patient has had a low-grade fever and growing pains in the lower legs. AP and lateral lower leg images were produced. In this scenario, the right lower leg images were normal so only left lower leg images are shown here.

1. How does the lower leg image demonstrate that this patient is young?

2. What anatomic structure relationships indicate true AP positioning?

Is the lower leg in a true AP position?

If not, what positioning error has occurred?

3. Due to the AP positioning error, what pathology is difficult to visualize?

4. On a lateral image at a 90-degree perspective, what pathology becomes more easily identifiable?

5. Did the radiographer select the correct exposure factors to demonstrate the pathology in this case?

If not, how should the exposure factors be adjusted?

6. What could the lucency be the result of?

7. What is the differential diagnosis?

An adult male patient entered the emergency department limping. He twisted his foot playing basketball. A routine foot series was performed and is presented here:

1. On the dorsoplantar projection, are any abnormalities noted?

Describe what is visualized.

2. Are the toes properly exposed?

What changes could be made to better demonstrate the toes?

3. The oblique projection demonstrates an abnormality at the base of the fifth metatarsal. What is it?

4. On the lateral projection, is the area of interest well demonstrated?

What might the radiographer do to improve this image?

5. This image series demonstrates the importance of what positioning rule?

6. What is the most common fracture of the foot?

An adult male patient was brought to the emergency department by ambulance stretcher following a motor vehicle collision. The patient was in a cervical collar for immobilization purposes. A routine trauma C-spine series was performed. The resident and radiologist considered the image results normal and "cleared" the patient from needing cervical spine precautions. The patient was scheduled for direct coronal images of the facial bones. The radiographer was uncomfortable in placing the patient into hyperextension without seeing the axial projections first. The following images were taken:

1. What structures demonstrate discontinuity? Which vertebra is fractured?

2. What is the name of this fracture?

3. By completing the axial projections first, did the radiographer practice outside his or her "scope of practice"?

4. If axial images are not ordered, can the radiographer add them to the scan series?

Note: CT scans of the spine are becoming more common in trauma cases for just this type of situation. Scanners are much more efficient, provide multiplanar images, and usually take less time than the plain trauma C-spine radiographic series.

SELF-TEST

Read each question carefully, then circle the best answer.

1. For patients with severe osteoporosis, how should the exposure factors be adjusted?
   a. Increase
   b. Decrease
   c. No change
   d. Increase exposure time

2. Osteopetrosis requires changes in the exposure factors. The radiographer should
   a. Increase exposure time
   b. No change
   c. decrease
   d. increase

3. The modality of choice to demonstrate cortical bone loss in osteoporosis is a(n)
   a. DEXA scan
   b. quantitative CT scan
   c. plain radiograph
   d. NM bone scan

4. The early stage of this disease process is seen as sharply demarcated radiolucency, which represents the destructive phase of
   a. Pott disease
   b. Paget disease
   c. gout
   d. osteomyelitis

5. Enchondromas are
   a. slow-growing benign cartilaginous tumors
   b. benign projections of bone with cartilaginous caps
   c. eccentric lucent lesions in the metaphysis
   d. well-circumscribed, extremely dense round lesions

6. An expansile lucent lesion with a thin sclerotic rim is a(n)
   a. osteoma
   b. bone island
   c. aneurysmal bone cyst
   d. unicameral bone cyst

7. What tumors arise in the medullary cavity of the small bones of the hands and feet?
   a. enchondromas
   b. endodermomas
   c. osteochondromas
   d. osteosarcomas

8. For osteoid osteoma, what modality is used to best demonstrate the nidus?
   a. CT
   b. MRI
   c. US
   d. radiography

9. The most sensitive imaging modality to demonstrate ischemic necrosis is
   a. CT
   b. NM
   c. MRI
   d. plain radiographs

10. Insufficient mineralization of the immature skeleton causing a cupped and frayed metaphysis in long bones is
    a. osteomalacia
    b. rickets
    c. osteoporosis
    d. Paget disease

11. A cotton-wool radiographic appearance is visualized in the reparative phase of
    a. Pott disease
    b. Paget disease
    c. multiple myeloma
    d. osteopetrosis

12. Which is the least sensitive modality to demonstrate osteomyelitis because of its inability to demonstrate early destruction?
    a. radiography
    b. CT
    c. MRI
    d. NM

13. Although the DEXA scan involves less radiation exposure for the patient, quantitative CT is one modality to demonstrate which disease?
    a. osteopetrosis
    b. osteoporosis
    c. osteomalacia
    d. osteoma

14. The spine consists of an anterior column and a posterior column. When both columns are disrupted, the injury is considered
    a. displaced
    b. stable
    c. undisplaced
    d. unstable

15. Which fracture is a transverse fracture at the base of the fifth metatarsal?
    a. Jones
    b. Pott
    c. boxer's
    d. Galeazzi

16. It is common in what type of fracture for the healing process to halt and the fragments to remain separate, creating a serious complication, possibly necrosis?
    a. scaphoid
    b. pathologic
    c. boxer's
    d. Jones

17. The malignant bone tumor most commonly found in the metaphysis of the knee is a(n)
    a. osteochondroma
    b. osteogenic sarcoma
    c. chondrosarcoma
    d. multiple myeloma

18. Which tumor has a classic radiographic appearance of an ill-defined permeative area of bone destruction involving a large central portion of the shaft of a long bone?
    a. Ewing sarcoma
    b. osteosarcoma
    c. chondrosarcoma
    d. osteoid osteoma

19. To evaluate and grade spondylolisthesis, the radiologist needs a(n)
    a. standing AP lumbar spine image
    b. oblique lumbar spine image
    c. lateral lumbar spine image
    d. standing lateral lumbar spine image

20. To diagnose spondylolysis, the routine images should include
    a. AP and lateral cervical spine images
    b. AP, oblique, and lateral cervical spine images
    c. AP and lateral lumbar spine images
    d. AP, oblique, and lateral lumbar spine images

21. To best demonstrate a herniation of an intervertebral disk requires which of the following procedures?
    a. CT myelogram
    b. PET body scan
    c. US of the spinal cord
    d. NM bone scan

22. Which fracture is a transverse fracture of the spine often associated with significant visceral injuries?
    a. seat belt
    b. hangman's
    c. clay shoveler's
    d. Jefferson

23. Ingestion of which substance is interchangeable with that of calcium in the body, causing dense transverse bands in the metaphysis?
    a. hypervitaminosis
    b. lead
    c. vitamin K
    d. increased caloric intake

24. To best image scoliosis, the patient should be
    a. recumbent bending away from the curvature
    b. recumbent prone
    c. standing with equal stance
    d. recumbent bending toward the curvature

5 Gastrointestinal System

OBJECTIVES

In addition to the objectives listed at the beginning of Chapter 5 in the textbook, the user should be able to:
1. Identify anatomic structures on diagrams and radiographs of the gastrointestinal system.
2. Describe the physiology of the gastrointestinal system.
3. Differentiate the pathologic disorders of the gastrointestinal system by defining the disease processes and their radiographic manifestations.
4. Determine changes in technical factors to obtain optimal-quality radiographs for patients with various underlying pathologic conditions.

EXERCISE 1: LABELING—ANATOMY

Identify the anatomic structures indicated by writing the correct name(s) in the space(s) provided.

A, Location of the digestive organs.

1 _____ _____

2 _____ _____   10 _____

3 _____ _____ _____

4 _____ _____   11 _____

5 _____ _____   12 _____
                                                               13 _____

6 _____ _____   14 _____

7 _____ _____   15 _____

8 _____ _____   16 _____

9 _____ _____   17 _____

                                                               18 _____

                                                               19 _____

(From Solomon P: *Introduction to human anatomy and physiology*, ed 4, St. Louis, 2016, Saunders.)

B, Stomach.

15 _____
14 _____
13 _____
12 _____
11 _____
10 _____
9 _____
8 _____
7 _____

S
R ⊕ L
I

1 _____
2 _____
3 _____
4 _____
5 _____
6 _____

(From Thibodeau GA, Patton KT: *Anatomy and physiology*, ed 6, St. Louis, 2007, Mosby.)

C, Divisions of the large intestine.

14 _____
13 _____
12 _____
11 _____
10 _____
9 _____
8 _____
7 _____
6 _____

S
R ⊕ L
I

1 _____
2 _____
3 _____
4 _____
5 _____

(From Mettler FA Jr: *Essentials of radiology*, ed 2, 2004, Elsevier.)

Chapter **5** **Gastrointestinal System**

D, Ducts that carry bile from the liver and gallbladder.

10 _____   11 _____

9 _____

8 _____

7 _____

6 _____

5 _____

1 _____

2 _____

3 _____

4 _____

S
R ✦ L
I

(From Thibodeau GA, Patton KT: *Anatomy and physiology*, ed 6, St. Louis, 2007, Mosby.)

EXERCISE 2: FILL IN THE BLANK—PHYSIOLOGY

Complete the following questions by writing the correct term(s) in the blank(s) provided.

1. The main function of the digestive system is to alter the _____ and _____ composition of food.

2. Altering the composition of food enables it to be _____ and _____ by body cells.

3. The two types of glands associated with changing the composition of food are _____ and _____.

4. Digestion begins in the _____ with _____.

5. Precise opening and closing of the esophageal sphincter requires coordination of many muscles for _____ to occur.

6. Acids and enzymes mix with gastric content, resulting in a milky-white _____.

7. Smooth muscle contractions that propel the gastric content through the digestive system are known as _____.

8. Fat digestion requires _____ to permit it to mix with water.

9. The pancreas produces enzymes for digestion of _____.

10. The completion of digestion means that the body can absorb nutrients through the _____ _____.

11. Four examples of fat-soluble vitamins are _____, _____, _____, and _____.

12. The pancreas secretes _____ and _____ to control the level of glucose in the circulating blood.

EXERCISE 3: FILL IN THE BLANK—GASTROINTESTINAL PATHOLOGY

Complete the following questions by writing the correct term(s) in the blank(s) provided.

1. In some cases of _____ _____, the upper and lower segments of the esophagus are blind pouches.

2. Double-contrast studies best demonstrate the superficial ulceration or erosions in the distal esophagus, which appear as streaks or dots of barium in _____ _____ disease.

3. Ingestion of _____ _____ produces acute inflammatory changes, including superficial to deep ulcerations.

4. _____ diverticula arise from the posterior wall of the upper esophagus, sometimes large enough to almost occlude the lumen.

5. The radiographic appearance of esophageal _____ is serpiginous thickening of folds resembling the beads of a rosary.

6. Free air in the mediastinum or periesophageal soft tissue on radiographs implies a possible _____ of the esophagus.

7. _____ occurs when the two muscular layers of the pylorus become hyperplastic and hypertrophic.

8. Irritants in the stomach, such as alcohol, corrosive agents, and infection, cause _____.

9. The enzyme _____ causes an inflammatory process to occur most often in the lesser curvature of the stomach, resulting in a(n) _____.

10. _____ disease of the small bowel usually involves the terminal ileum and is a granulomatous inflammatory process.

11. Patients with complete _____ obstruction of the small bowel demonstrate little or no gas in the colon.

12. The small bowel and large bowel appear uniformly dilated with no demonstrable point of obstruction on the abdominal radiographs in a patient with a(n)_____ _____.

13. An appendicolith may cause gangrene or perforation, resulting in _____.

14. Patients with ulcerative colitis are 10 times more frequently affected by _____ of the colon.

15. A loss of haustral markings and deep ulcers outlined by intraluminal gas may indicate _____ _____.

16. A sessile polyp demonstrating growth with an irregular or lobulated surface on sequential examinations is indicative of _____ _____.

17. Inflammation of the gallbladder, usually after obstruction of the cystic duct by a gallstone, is _____ _____.

18. Calcification of the wall of the gallbladder is referred to as a _____ gallbladder, indicating the possibility of _____.

19. Diffuse or focal enlargement of the gland with obscured soft tissue on _____ images is acute pancreatitis.

20. Pancreatic calcifications are the _____ finding in chronic pancreatitis.

21. The most common cause of pneumoperitoneum is associated with _____ of an _____.

22. The viral infection most prevalent in inflammatory disease of the liver is _____.

23. Hepatitis _____ virus is contracted by exposure to contaminated blood or blood products, or through sexual contact.

EXERCISE 4: MATCHING—ANATOMY AND PHYSIOLOGY

Match each of the following terms with the correct definition by placing the letter of the best answer in the space provided. Each question has only one correct answer. Please note that there are more terms than definitions.

1. _____ bile is an example

2. _____ chewing

3. _____ consists of salts, cholesterol, and bilirubin

4. _____ excess glucose stored in the body

5. _____ fingerlike projections in the small bowel

6. _____ helps move the chyme through the digestive tract

7. _____ milky-white product found in the stomach

8. _____ produces an emulsifier

9. _____ produces enzymes to aid in digestion of proteins

10. _____ produces hydrochloric acid and the proteolytic enzyme pepsin

11. _____ stores bile for use by the digestive system

12. _____ swallowing

A. bile

B. chyme

C. constipation

D. deglutition

E. diarrhea

F. emulsifier

G. gallbladder

H. glycogen

I. liver

J. mastication

K. pancreas

L. peristalsis

M. stomach

N. villi

Match each of the following terms with the correct definition by placing the letter of the best answer in the space provided. Each question has only one correct answer. Please note that there are more terms than definitions.

1. _____ any symptomatic condition or structural changes due to reflux of stomach content into the esophagus

2. _____ complete rupture of the esophageal wall

3. _____ dilated veins in the esophageal wall

4. _____ disease that appears as a persistent collection of barium surrounded by a halo of edema

5. _____ disease in which the edematous and thickened pylorus may be palpated and is described as a mobile, hard "olive"

6. _____ disorder in which the esophageal lumen does not develop separately from the trachea

7. _____ fungus or virus causing a cobblestone pattern caused by deep ulcerations and sloughing of the mucosa

8. _____ incomplete relaxation of the lower esophageal sphincter causing esophageal dilatation

9. _____ inflammation of the stomach manifesting as an abnormal surface pattern in the gastric mucosa

10. _____ inflammatory process of the stomach and duodenum caused by the action of acid

11. _____ most common manifestation of peptic ulcer disease

12. _____ most often occurs in the distal stomach and is of glandular origin

13. _____ a tumor that most often is of squamous cell type and occurs at the esophagogastric junction

14. _____ condition in which much of the stomach lies within the thoracic cavity

15. _____ disorder in which normal squamous lining is destroyed and replaced with columnar epithelium

16. _____ outpouching herniating through the muscular layer of the esophagus

17. _____ severe mucosal atrophy causing thinning or an absence of mucosal folds

A. achalasia

B. acute gastritis

C. Barrett esophagus

D. chronic atrophic gastritis

E. diverticula

F. duodenal ulcer

G. esophageal carcinoma

H. esophageal varices

I. foreign bodies

J. gastric ulcer

K. gastroesophageal reflux disease (GERD)

L. hiatal hernia

M. infectious esophagitis

N. peptic ulcer

O. perforation

P. pyloric stenosis

Q. stomach cancer

R. tracheoesophageal fistula

Match each of the following terms with the correct definition by placing the letter of the best answer in the space provided. Each question has only one correct answer. Please note that there are more terms than definitions.

1. _____ an inflammatory process usually of the proximal colon involving multiple noncontiguous segments (skip lesions)

2. _____ caused by previous surgery, peritonitis, or external hernias

3. _____ chronic granulomatous inflammatory disorder of unknown cause

4. _____ disorder of intestinal motility in which fluid and gas do not progress normally

5. _____ most common cause of bowel obstruction in children, caused by telescoping of the bowel into itself

6. _____ necrosing inflammation in the outpouchings representing acquired herniation

7. _____ neoplastic growth of which about half the cases occur in the rectum and sigmoid, most often in older men

8. _____ one of two inflammatory processes of unknown cause that primarily affect young adults

9. _____ outpouching representing acquired herniations of mucosa and submucosa through weak points in the muscular layer

10. _____ perforation permitting fecal material to enter the peritoneum, causing general peritonitis if not treated

11. _____ several conditions altering intestinal motility, usually functional disorders causing constipation or diarrhea (spastic colitis)

12. _____ twisting of the bowel on itself that leads to intestinal obstruction

A. adynamic ileus

B. appendicitis

C. carcinoma of the small bowel

D. Crohn colitis

E. Crohn disease

F. colonic carcinoma

G. diverticulitis

H. diverticulosis

I. intussusception

J. irritable bowel syndrome

K. ischemic colitis

L. mechanical bowel obstruction

M. polyps

N. small bowel obstruction

O. ulcerative colitis

P. volvulus

EXERCISE 7: MATCHING—BILIARY AND PANCREATIC PATHOLOGY

Match each of the following terms with the correct definition by placing the letter of the best answer in the space provided. Each question has only one correct answer. Please note that there are more terms than definitions.

1. _____ cholesterol and pigment stones

2. _____ chronic process of destruction of liver cells and structure causing end-stage liver disease

3. _____ extensive calcification in the wall of the gallbladder

4. _____ gas-forming organisms that are facilitated by stasis and ischemia due to cystic duct obstruction

5. _____ loculated fluid collections resulting from the process associated with acute pancreatitis

6. _____ most common neoplastic process involving the liver

7. _____ neoplastic process occurring commonly in the head of the pancreas and causing the gland to have an irregular contour and semisolid pattern on the sonogram

8. _____ primary liver cancer

9. _____ disorder in which protein- and lipid-digesting enzymes become activated within the pancreas, causing the organ to ingest itself

10. _____ sudden attack of inflammation of the gallbladder

A. acute cholecystitis

B. acute pancreatitis

C. cholelithiasis

D. chronic pancreatitis

E. cirrhosis

F. emphysematous cholecystitis

G. hepatic metastasis

H. hepatitis

I. hepatocellular carcinoma

J. pancreatic adenocarcinoma

K. porcelain gallbladder

L. pseudocyst

EXERCISE 8: MULTIPLE CHOICE

Circle the best answer for each of the following multiple choice questions.

1. In type II tracheoesophageal fistulas, the upper segment _____ and the lower segment _____.
   a. ends in a blind pouch; also ends in a blind pouch
   b. communicates with the trachea; ends in a blind pouch
   c. ends in a blind pouch; attaches to the trachea
   d. ends in a blind pouch; ends in a blind pouch with both connecting to the trachea

2. The condition related to severe reflux esophagitis in which the normal squamous lining of the lower esophagus is destroyed and replaced with columnar epithelium is known as
   a. Barrett esophagus
   b. esophageal cancer
   c. esophagitis
   d. gastroesophageal reflux

3. Mucosal and intramural inflammation of acute esophagitis may lead to pronounced fibrosis and stricture formation due to
   a. the ingestion of corrosive agents
   b. a herpes virus
   c. a fungal infection
   d. a polypoid mass

4. Irregularity of the esophageal wall indicating mucosal destruction possibly encircling the lumen is the radiographic appearance of
   a. gastroesophageal reflux
   b. esophagitis
   c. Barrett esophagus
   d. esophageal cancer

5. The esophagus and stomach are distinguished by the difference in the mucosal folds; demonstration of the stomach in the thoracic cavity is a case of
   a. Barrett esophagus
   b. esophagitis
   c. gastric reflux
   d. hiatal hernia

6. A functional obstruction of the distal esophagus resulting from incomplete relaxation of the lower esophageal sphincter is
   a. achalasia
   b. Barrett disease
   c. hiatal hernia
   d. due to ingestion of corrosive agents

7. Nonerosive or _____ gastritis refers to mucosal atrophy causing a thinning and absence of mucosal folds in the stomach.
   a. alcoholic
   b. bacterial
   c. chronic
   d. corrosive

8. The radiographic appearance of an ulcer causes
   a. a bald appearance due to the lack of mucosal folds
   b. thickened gastric walls causing a stricture
   c. a rounded or linear collection of contrast material surrounded by lucent folds
   d. infiltration of the gastric wall that produces diffuse thickening, narrowing, and stomach wall fixation

9. To demonstrate air-fluid levels in the abdomen, the technologist uses
   a. a horizontal beam on the upright image
   b. a perpendicular beam on the lateral decubitus image
   c. a perpendicular beam to the semierect patient
   d. either a or b

10. The loss of motility in the small bowel is referred to as
    a. adynamic ileus
    b. mechanical bowel obstruction
    c. intussusception
    d. herniation

11. A "doughnut-shaped" lesion on a transverse sonogram of the intestine is suspicious of a(n)
    a. hernia
    b. intussusception
    c. volvulus
    d. adynamic ileus

12. In diverticulosis, the diverticula appear radiographically as
    a. round or oval outpouchings beyond the confines of the lumen
    b. round or oval outpouchings with extravasation indicating perforation
    c. inward extensions of the mucosal wall
    d. deep ulcers outlined by intraluminal gas

13. Discrete erosions appearing as punctate collections with a surrounding thin halo of edema are the earliest radiographic findings in
    a. colon cancer
    b. Crohn colitis
    c. diverticulitis
    d. ulcerative colitis

14. Fine superficial ulcerations caused by inflammatory edema of the mucosa are indicative of
    a. Crohn colitis
    b. diverticulitis
    c. ulcerative colitis
    d. ischemic colitis

15. The pathognomonic sign of a kidney-shaped mass (twisted bowel) with a thickened and twisted mesentery is suspicious for
    a. colon cancer
    b. cecal volvulus
    c. sigmoid volvulus
    d. hemorrhoid

16. The modality of choice to demonstrate gallstones is
    a. US
    b. CT
    c. MRI
    d. kidney-ureter-bladder (KUB) radiograph

17. Large amounts of fat in the liver seen on CT or US images are suggestive of
    a. cirrhosis
    b. hepatocellular carcinoma
    c. hepatic metastasis
    d. an overweight patient

18. On US, an echo-free cystic structure with a sharp posterior wall and echogenic areas representing septations suggest
    a. pancreatic carcinoma
    b. chronic pancreatitis
    c. acute pancreatitis
    d. pancreatic pseudocyst

Chapter **5** **Gastrointestinal System**

19. Gas appearing as a sickle-shaped lucency on an abdominal image requires upright patient positioning and a horizontal beam. If the patient is unable to stand, the technologist should complete a
    a. right lateral decubitus image
    b. left lateral decubitus image
    c. semiupright KUB radiograph with the beam perpendicular to the patient
    d. KUB radiograph

20. CT best demonstrates blunt abdominal trauma for splenic laceration (the hematoma) as
    a. a crescentic collection
    b. focal enlargement
    c. a sickle-shaped lucency
    d. splenomegaly

EXERCISE 9: CASE STUDIES

The problems described in the following case studies required imaging of the gastrointestinal system. After each scenario, the image(s) are presented, and you are asked to answer questions. Using your knowledge of imaging pathology, apply exposure factors and positioning criteria to answer the questions.

CASE STUDY 1

A 2-day-old infant arrives in the radiology department for an esophagram. The infant is not thriving and has not fed since birth. The following anteroposterior and lateral images were produced as part of the fluoroscopic procedure:

1. Does the technologist ask the parents to assist during the fluoroscopic procedure?

2. Barium sulfate is the contrast medium of choice. How does the radiographer prepare this agent?

3. On the images shown, what device is being used to inject the contrast agent?

4. The contrast agent is filling what anatomic structure?

5. What esophageal disorder are the images demonstrating?

CASE STUDY 2

A 46-year-old patient enters the radiography department with an order for a small bowel series. The patient is experiencing abdominal cramping. A small bowel procedure was performed and the following images were presented:

Chapter **5** **Gastrointestinal System**

1. What causes pipelike narrowing in the small bowel?

2. The images demonstrate the pipelike narrowing referred to as what sign?

3. When the lesions are seen with normal small bowel separation, they are referred to as what?

4. The combination of these signs is referred to as which disorder?

5. The radiologist has a lead glove on and is pressing on the abdomen. Why?

6. If the lesions progress, the hallmark of this disease will occur. It is:

A 7-month-old boy was brought to the emergency department. The history involved continued crying for the last 12 hours. A routine barium enema study was performed and is shown here:

1. On image A, the bowel has a coiled-spring appearance. What is this appearance suggestive of?

2. Describe this disease process and why the coiled-spring appearance occurs.

3. What has started to occur on image B?

4. When a barium enema is performed, where should the enema bag be?

   Why is this especially important?

5. The preceding image demonstrates what has occurred?

6. In this case, would the barium enema study be considered diagnostic and/or therapeutic?

A 6-year-old patient was brought to the emergency department with chest and abdominal pain. A routine chest series was performed. The following is the posteroanterior upright chest image presented for evaluation:

1. What structures demonstrate that upright positioning was used as described by the labeling?

2. How long does the patient have to be in the upright position for air-fluid levels to become evident?

Chapter **5 Gastrointestinal System**

3. To ensure that adequate time passes before the upright image is completed, what is the first step the technologist should perform in this procedure?

4. If the patient arrives in the department in a wheelchair for recumbent and upright images of the chest and abdomen, which image(s) should be completed first? Why?

5. Is any free air demonstrated on this image? If so, where is it located?

6. What condition does this patient have?

7. If an upright position is not possible, the technologist should perform what alternate projection?

SELF-TEST

Read each question carefully, then circle the best answer.

1. Regional enteritis is also called
   a. Barrett disease
   b. Cushing disease
   c. Crohn disease
   d. Zollinger-Ellison disease

2. What disease is known for demonstrating the pathologic disorder known as the string sign?
   a. Crohn disease
   b. esophageal varices
   c. paralytic ileus
   d. ulcerative colitis

3. The term for outpouchings along the walls of the bowel lumen is
   a. ulcer
   b. diverticula
   c. polyp
   d. fibrosis

4. The condition involving large amounts of air in dilated loops of large and small bowel is referred to as
   a. colonic ileus
   b. ischemic ileus
   c. localized ileus
   d. adynamic ileus

5. The classic appearance of annular carcinoma of the colon is a(n)
   a. apple core
   b. bird's nest
   c. eggshell
   d. ground glass

6. Varicose veins of the rectum are
   a. diverticula
   b. fibroids
   c. hemorrhoids
   d. polyps

7. The condition in which the bowel telescopes into itself is
   a. herniation
   b. ileus
   c. intussusception
   d. volvulus

8. The stepladder sign is indicative of
   a. adynamic ileus
   b. paralytic ileus
   c. regional enteritis
   d. small bowel obstruction

9. The major cause of cirrhosis in the United States and Europe is
   a. alcoholism
   b. elevated blood cholesterol
   c. hepatitis
   d. overweight populations

10. The most common viral inflammatory disease of the liver is
    a. HIV
    b. AIDS
    c. toxoid exposure
    d. hepatitis

11. The form of hepatitis contracted by exposure to contaminated blood products or through sexual contact is
    a. hepatitis A
    b. hepatitis B
    c. hepatitis C
    d. hepatitis E

12. If the patient is too ill to stand, what position should the patient be placed in to demonstrate pneumoperitoneum?
    a. right lateral decubitus, patient on the right side
    b. right lateral decubitus, patient on the left side
    c. left lateral decubitus, patient on the right side
    d. left lateral decubitus, patient on the left side

13. Twisting of the bowel upon itself is
    a. adynamic ileus
    b. volvulus
    c. intussusception
    d. regional enteritis

14. A colonic intussusception can sometimes be reduced by which radiographic procedure or modality?
    a. CT
    b. small bowel series
    c. barium enema
    d. enteroclysis

15. The medical term denoting difficulty swallowing is
    a. deglutition
    b. dysphagia
    c. dyspnea
    d. mastication

16. An abnormal connection between the esophagus and trachea is called a(n)
    a. fistula
    b. malformation
    c. achalasia
    d. atresia

17. Little or no gas seen in the small bowel is indication of
    a. colonic ileus
    b. mechanical bowel obstruction
    c. paralytic bowel obstruction
    d. paralytic ileus

18. A loss of haustral markings and deep ulcerations surrounded by intraluminal gas is indicative of
    a. infectious colitis
    b. ischemic colitis
    c. regional colitis
    d. ulcerative colitis

19. Malignant polyps tend to be
    a. irregular and pedunculated
    b. irregular and sessile
    c. smooth and pedunculated
    d. smooth and sessile

20. Enzymes that aid in the digestion of proteins are produced by the
    a. duodenal bulb
    b. liver
    c. pancreas
    d. stomach

21. The milky-white product found in the stomach is
    a. chyme
    b. hydrochloric acid
    c. gastric enzymes
    d. bile

22. Any symptomatic condition or structural changes caused by reflux of stomach content into the esophagus is
    a. hiatal hernia
    b. gastric ulcer
    c. GERD
    d. esophageal carcinoma

23. Inflammation of the stomach manifesting as an abnormal surface pattern in the gastric mucosa is suggestive of
    a. acute gastritis
    b. chronic atrophic gastritis
    c. peptic ulcer
    d. duodenal ulcer

24. An outpouching of the posterior wall of the esophagus is considered
    a. a traction diverticulum
    b. Zenker diverticulum
    c. an esophageal polyp
    d. Mallory-Weiss syndrome

25. The condition in which cholesterol and pigment sediment blocks the common bile duct, causing an inflammatory attack, is known as
    a. cholelithiasis
    b. acute cholecystitis
    c. chronic cholecystitis
    d. acute pancreatitis

26. A functional obstruction of the distal esophagus resulting from incomplete relaxation of the lower esophageal sphincter is
    a. achalasia
    b. Barrett disease
    c. hiatal hernia
    d. due to ingestion of corrosive agents

27. A doughnut-shaped lesion on a transverse sonogram of the intestine is suspicious for
    a. adynamic ileus
    b. hernia
    c. intussusception
    d. volvulus

6 | Urinary System

OBJECTIVES

In addition to the objectives listed at the beginning of Chapter 6 in the textbook, the user should be able to:
1. Identify anatomic structures on diagrams and radiographs of the urinary system.
2. Describe the physiology of the urinary system.
3. Differentiate the pathologic disorders of the urinary system by defining the disease processes and their radiographic manifestations.
4. Determine changes in technical factors to obtain optimal-quality radiographs for patients with various underlying pathologic conditions.

EXERCISE 1: LABELING—ANATOMY

Identify the anatomic structures indicated by writing the correct names in the spaces provided.

A, Location of the urinary system.

11 _____

10 _____

9 _____

8 _____

7 _____

1 _____

2 _____

3 _____

4 _____

5 _____

6 _____

S
R — L
I

(From Abrahams P, Hutchings RT, Marks SC: *McMinn's color atlas of human anatomy*, ed 4, St. Louis, 1999, Mosby.)

B, Internal structure of the kidney.

Interlobular arteries

Renal column

1 _____

2 _____

11 _____

3 _____

10 _____

4 _____

9 _____

8 _____

7 _____

5 _____

6 _____

(From Brundage DJ: *Renal disorders*, St. Louis, 1992, Mosby.)

C, Structure and location of the male urinary bladder.

Ureter

1 _____

2 _____

3 _____

10 _____

4 _____

9 _____

5 _____

8 _____

6 _____

7 _____

Bulbourethral gland

(From Thibodeau GA, Patton KT: *Anatomy and physiology*, ed 7, St. Louis, 2010, Mosby.)

EXERCISE 2: FILL IN THE BLANK—ANATOMY AND PHYSIOLOGY

Complete the following questions by writing the correct term(s) in the blank(s) provided.

1. The main function of the kidney is to filter the _____ from the blood and _____ water and nutrients, and _____ excess substances.

2. The functional unit of the kidney is the _____.

3. The formation of urine begins in the _____.

4. The _____ _____ _____ is where virtually all nutrients are reabsorbed into the blood capillaries.

5. The three structures that make up the complex structure known as the loop of Henle are the _____, _____, and _____.

6. The kidney helps to maintain _____ balance and _____ balance of blood and body fluids.

7. The urine passes from the collecting tubules, which open into the _____.

8. From the calyces, the urine passes into the _____.

9. The bladder acts as a _____ for urine until it leaves the body.

10. On the posterior aspect of the bladder, there are three openings where the _____, _____, and _____ enter or exit.

11. The triangle-shaped area on the floor of the bladder is called the _____.

12. The bladder, when full, is stimulated by the autonomic nervous system to produce a sensation to _____ or _____.

13. When the bladder contracts, the urine travels through the _____, exiting the body.

14. A complicated sequence of bladder contractions and relaxation of the _____ _____ permits the bladder to expel urine from the body through the urethra.

15. Involuntary emptying of the bladder is referred to as _____.

EXERCISE 3: FILL IN THE BLANK—URINARY PATHOLOGY

Complete the following questions by writing the correct term(s) in the blank(s) provided.

1. The phenomenon in which one kidney must perform the function normally carried out by two kidneys is called _____ _____.

2. The kidney's position in relation to the psoas muscle on radiographs appears elongated or foreshortened in cases in which the kidney has _____.

3. On US images, a _____ appears as a round, cyst-like mass within the bladder, contiguous with a dilated ureter.

4. The term for more than one ureter or renal pelvis is _____.

5. Ultrasound demonstrates the lower poles of the kidney fused, resulting in a _____ _____.

6. In chronic _____, the kidneys are bilaterally smaller with normal contours.

7. The spread of _____ to the renal pyramid causes an ulcerative, destructive process with irregularity and enlargement of the calyces.

8. The necrotic process in _____ _____ causes cavitations in the central portion of the papillae.

9. Noncontrast computed tomography (CT) is the safest method to demonstrate _____ _____.

10. The renal calculus that fills the renal calyces and pelvis is called a _____ calculus.

11. When a blockage in the ureter occurs above the bladder, it may cause a _____.

12. The four normal points of narrowing that are common sites of obstruction in the urinary system are the _____, _____, _____, and _____.

13. The most common unifocal mass of the kidney is a _____.

14. A multilobulated contour caused by multiple cysts in the parenchyma is _____ _____ disease.

15. The triad of symptoms in renal carcinoma consists of _____, _____, and _____.

16. Renal enlargement or localized bulging with elongation of adjacent calyces in an excretory urogram is suggestive of _____ _____.

17. _____ _____ is the most common abdominal neoplasm of infancy and childhood that arises from embryonic renal tissue, may be bilateral, and tends to become very large and appear as a palpable mass.

18. A plain radiograph showing punctate, coarse, or linear calcifications, usually on the periphery of the bladder, is suggestive of _____.

19. _____ _____ _____ occurs most frequently in children who are severely dehydrated and most often is a complication of another renal disease in adults.

20. _____ _____ _____ refers to a rapid deterioration in kidney function that results in the accumulation of nitrogen-containing wastes in the blood, causing an odor of urine-like or "fishy" breath.

EXERCISE 4: MATCHING—ANATOMY AND PHYSIOLOGY

Match each of the following terms with the correct definition by placing the letter of the best answer in the space provided. Each question has only one correct answer. Please note that there are more terms than definitions.

1. _____ area of kidney where the blood vessels, renal pelvis, and nerves enter and exit the kidney

2. _____ carries the urine from the kidney to the bladder

3. _____ complex structure consisting of a descending limb, loop, and ascending limb

4. _____ cup-shaped top of a nephron that surrounds the glomerulus

5. _____ muscular structure on the posterior aspect of the bladder

6. _____ process of voiding

7. _____ provides the path for urine to exit the body

8. _____ stores urine before entrance into the renal pelvis

9. _____ term describing the process by which the loop of Henle keeps a balance of salts in the body

10. _____ tuft of capillaries with very thin walls and a large surface area

11. _____ uncontrolled response of voiding

12. _____ urine passes into the papillae through this structure

A. acid-base balance

B. Bowman's capsule

C. collecting tubules

D. electrolyte balance

E. glomerulus

F. hilum

G. incontinence

H. loop of Henle

I. major calyces

J. micturition

K. proximal convoluted tubule

L. renal pelvis

M. trigone

N. ureter

O. urethra

Chapter **6 Urinary System**

EXERCISE 5: MATCHING—URINARY PATHOLOGY

Match each of the following terms with the correct definition by placing the letter of the best answer in the space provided. Each question has only one correct answer. Please note that there are more terms than definitions.

1. _____ 80% of these structures contain enough calcium to be radiopaque

2. _____ a third kidney

3. _____ cystic dilatation of the distal ureter

4. _____ destructive process involving the medullary papillae and the terminal renal pyramids

5. _____ dilatation of the renal pelvicalyceal area

6. _____ dilatation of the ureter

7. _____ ectopic kidney found in the pelvis

8. _____ evidence of a solitary kidney

9. _____ extension of a clot from the inferior vena cava

10. _____ fingerlike projections into the lumen of the bladder

11. _____ fluid-filled unilocular mass

12. _____ inflammation of the urinary bladder

13. _____ inflammatory process involving the tufts of the capillaries that filter the blood

14. _____ lesion arising from embryonic renal tissue most commonly found in infants and during childhood

15. _____ fusion of the lower poles of the left and right kidneys

16. _____ most common renal neoplasm, also known as a hypernephroma

17. _____ multiple cysts of varying sizes causing progressive renal impairment

18. _____ pyogenic bacteria causing inflammation of the kidney and renal pelvis

19. _____ results in a condition called uremia, an accumulation of excessive blood levels of urea and creatinine

20. _____ thin transverse membrane in the urethra preventing micturition

A. acute renal failure

B. bladder carcinoma

C. chronic renal failure

D. cystitis

E. glomerulonephritis

F. horseshoe kidney

G. hydronephrosis

H. hydroureter

I. papillary necrosis

J. polycystic kidney

K. positioning anomaly

L. posterior urethral valves

M. pyelonephritis

N. renal agenesis

O. renal carcinoma

P. renal cyst

Q. renal vein thrombus

R. supernumerary kidney

S. ureterocele

T. urinary calculi

U. Wilms tumor

EXERCISE 6: MULTIPLE CHOICE

Circle the best answer for each of the following multiple choice questions.

1. A miniature replica of a normal kidney with good function is a
   a. compensatory kidney
   b. hypoplastic kidney
   c. supernumerary kidney
   d. hyperplastic kidney

2. A kidney that is not located in the retroperitoneal space adjacent to the psoas muscle is considered
   a. an ectopic kidney
   b. a compensatory kidney
   c. a hypertrophic kidney
   d. a horseshoe kidney

3. The modality that demonstrates the fused inferior poles of the kidneys without radiation exposure is
   a. CT
   b. ultrasound (US)
   c. magnetic resonance imaging (MRI)
   d. intravenous urography (IVU)

4. The _____ is a thin membrane that prevents normal urine flow.
   a. posterior urethral valve
   b. ureteropelvic junction
   c. ureterovesical junction
   d. ureterocele

5. A horseshoe kidney
   a. is lower-pole parenchymal fusion
   b. indicates a supernumerary kidney
   c. is a duplication of the ureters and renal pelvis
   d. indicates an out-of-position kidney

6. A dilatation of the ureter at the ureterovesical junction is a
   a. ureterocele
   b. urethral valve
   c. posterior urethral valve
   d. duplicated renal pelvis

7. Chronic pyelonephritis causes the kidneys to
   a. diminish in size
   b. have irregular contours and clubbing of the calyces
   c. produce radiolucent gas shadows within and around the kidney
   d. necrose in the central portion of the papillae

8. Small granulomas scattered in the cortices of the kidney occurs in the hematogenous spread of
   a. glomerulonephritis
   b. nephritis
   c. polynephritis
   d. tuberculosis

9. Gas-forming bacteria appearing as a lucent ring outlining all or part of the bladder on plain radiographs are suggestive of
   a. emphysematous cystitis
   b. emphysematous pyelonephritis
   c. tuberculosis
   d. urinary calculi

10. The composition of urinary calculi can be
    a. calcium
    b. oxalates
    c. sodium
    d. a or b

11. The minuscule deposits of calcium within the renal parenchyma are
    a. urinary calculi
    b. renal calculi
    c. nephrocalcinosis
    d. tuberculosis

12. Hydronephrosis is commonly caused by
    a. a kidney stone
    b. sodium carbonate
    c. lack of peristalsis
    d. an overload of potassium

13. The modality or procedure of choice to differentiate a fluid-filled simple cyst from a solid mass is
    a. CT
    b. excretory urography
    c. kidney-ureter-bladder (KUB) radiograph
    d. US

14. An inherited disorder in which multiple cysts of varying size cause lobulated enlargement of the kidneys and progressive renal impairment is
    a. hypernephroma
    b. polycystic disease
    c. Wilms tumor
    d. renal carcinoma

15. A renal carcinoma demonstrates as a solid mass with numerous internal echoes and no evidence of acoustic enhancement when imaged with
    a. CT
    b. excretory urography
    c. MRI
    d. US

16. In acute renal failure, US demonstrates
    a. atrophic kidneys
    b. intrarenal or perirenal infection
    c. post-obstructive hypernephrosis
    d. renal function

17. Polypoid defects and bladder wall thickening are indicative of
    a. hypernephroma
    b. nephroblastoma
    c. bladder carcinoma
    d. cystitis

18. A highly malignant renal tumor most common in infancy and childhood is
    a. hypernephroma
    b. renal carcinoma
    c. Wilms tumor
    d. polycystic disease

EXERCISE 7: CASE STUDIES

The problems described in the following case studies required imaging of the urinary system. After each scenario, the images are presented, and you will be asked to answer questions. Using your knowledge of imaging pathology, apply exposure factors and positioning criteria to answer the questions.

CASE STUDY 1

A stabbing victim arrives in the emergency department (ED) with a puncture wound on the left posterior abdomen. The following contrast-enhanced CT images were obtained as part of the ED workup.

1. On CT scans, the normal kidney has smooth contours and lies lateral and anterior to the psoas muscle (image A). What differences are apparent on the scan in image B?

2. Does the contrast enhancement help delineate and differentiate the hematoma from the renal tissue? How?

3. What is the differential diagnosis for this appearance?

Part 2 of this case study involves a patient who experienced blunt-force trauma to the back. The CT examination was completed at 5-mm increments with contrast enhancement, and the following images were obtained:

4. In image A, there appears to be pressure moving the liver anteriorly from a mass effect located posterior to the liver. Given the patient history, what does the mass possibly represent?

5. On image B, the region of the mass is associated with which anatomic structure?

6. What is the differential diagnosis for this appearance?

Chapter 6 Urinary System

A patient enters the radiography department with an order for an excretory urogram. The patient is experiencing left flank pain and has hematuria. An IVU was performed, with the following initial images obtained:

SCOUT

1. The protocol for excretory urography requires a "scout" image before the contrast portion of the examination is begun. Of what importance is the preceding image?

2. Is any pathology demonstrated on the scout image?

3. Once the contrast is injected, what will the pathology demonstrate?

Part 2 of this case study involves the following scout image in another patient, which was also the initial image for an excretory urogram and has been cropped to include only the pelvis:

4. In this case, what pathology is demonstrated?

5. When contrast material from the IVU enters the bladder, will the pathology be evident?

6. What is the differential diagnosis?

An 83-year-old man entered the radiology department for a scheduled cystogram. The clinical findings indicated the possibility of the bladder tracking through the inguinal canal; a cystogram was the procedure of choice to rule out this diagnosis. A routine cystogram was performed, and the following images were obtained:

1. The tube entering the bladder represents the _____.

2. What does image A demonstrate?

3. Does this image demonstrate any possible pathology?

4. On the oblique view shown in image A of the preceding image, where is the contrast material located?

5. The lateral image (image B) was taken to provide what additional information?

6. What pathologic conditions can describe the appearance of these images?

Read each question carefully, then circle the best answer.

1. To ensure that the diagnosis is renal agenesis, the best modality or image to demonstrate the abdomen is
   a. KUB radiograph
   b. IVU
   c. CT
   d. US

2. An abnormal position of the kidney in relationship to the psoas muscle in the retroperitoneal location is considered
   a. ectopic
   b. to indicate malrotation
   c. hypertrophic
   d. hypoplastic

3. When IVU demonstrates two ureters exiting from one kidney, what term is used to describe the condition?
   a. duplication
   b. fused
   c. ectopic
   d. malrotation

4. A second kidney found in the pelvis or thoracic cavity is considered a(n)
   a. ectopic kidney
   b. duplicated kidney
   c. rotated kidney
   d. fused kidney

5. A transverse membrane in the urethra demonstrates as a stricture or narrowing in a
   a. ureterocele
   b. supernumerary kidney
   c. posterior urethral valve
   d. duplicated renal pelvis

6. On CT urography, a characteristic ring of contrast material surrounds a triangular lucent filling defect, representing the sloughed tissue in
   a. tuberculosis
   b. papillary necrosis
   c. glomerulonephritis
   d. pyelonephritis

7. Irregularity of the bladder wall and a diminished size are indicative of
   a. nephritis
   b. cystitis
   c. bladder carcinoma
   d. tuberculosis

8. Hydroureter and hydronephrosis are complications of
   a. infection in the renal cortices
   b. nephrocalcinosis
   c. obstruction due to a ureteral calculus
   d. papillary necrosis

9. Hydronephrosis can be caused by
   a. polycystic kidney disease
   b. reflux
   c. obstruction
   d. all of the above

10. Which modality or procedure best detects mass effects, stones, and other causes of renal obstruction?
    a. CT
    b. excretory urography
    c. cystogram
    d. US

11. Sonography demonstrates hydronephrosis as
    a. thickened cortices
    b. an echogenic region with acoustic shadowing
    c. echo-free sacs
    d. shadowing and swollen pyramids

12. The most common unifocal masses of the kidney that are fluid filled and usually unilocular is
    a. renal cyst
    b. renal carcinoma
    c. Wilms tumor
    d. hypernephroma

13. To distinguish fluid-filled from solid lesions, the modality or procedure of choice is
    a. radiography, KUB image
    b. CT
    c. US
    d. radiography, excretory urography

14. Polycystic kidney disease consists of
    a. a fluid-filled cyst
    b. multiple cysts of varying sizes
    c. an embryonic renal mass
    d. a cyst with calcification

15. The most accurate imaging modality or procedure for detecting local and regional spread of renal cell carcinoma is
    a. CT
    b. US
    c. radiography, excretory urography
    d. radiography, KUB image

16. The condition that appears as a round, cyst-like mass within the bladder, contiguous with a dilated ureter, is
    a. posterior urethral valve
    b. renal carcinoma
    c. renal cyst
    d. ureteroceles

17. Rapid deterioration in kidney function resulting in an accumulation of waste in the blood is suggestive of
    a. acute renal failure
    b. chronic renal failure
    c. nephrocalcinosis
    d. urinary calculus

18. The symptom triad consisting of hematuria, flank pain, and, possibly, a palpable mass, defines
    a. Wilms tumor
    b. renal carcinoma
    c. hyperplasia
    d. hyponephroma

19. Underlying causes for what condition include bilateral renal stenosis, bilateral ureteral obstruction, and intrinsic renal disorders?
    a. chronic renal failure
    b. renal carcinoma
    c. papillary necrosis
    d. glomerulonephritis

20. A condition that results in failure to clear nitrogen-containing wastes adequately from circulation leading to the accumulation of excessive blood levels of urea and creatinine in the blood is
    a. electrolyte imbalance
    b. uremia
    c. potassium imbalance
    d. sodium chloride imbalance

7 Cardiovascular System

OBJECTIVES

In addition to the objectives listed at the beginning of Chapter 7 in the textbook, the user should be able to:
1. Identify anatomic structures on diagrams and radiographs of the cardiovascular system.
2. Describe the physiology of the cardiovascular system.
3. Differentiate the pathologic disorders of the cardiovascular system by defining the disease processes and their radiographic manifestations.
4. Determine changes in technical factors to obtain optimal-quality radiographs for patients with various underlying pathologic conditions.

EXERCISE 1: LABELING—ANATOMY

Identify the anatomic structures indicated by writing the correct name in the space provided.

A, Conduction system of the heart and vascular anatomy.

(From Thibodeau GA, Patton KT: *Anatomy and physiology*, ed 6, St. Louis, 2007, Mosby.)

B, Structure of the heart valves.

Skeleton of heart, including
fibrous rings around valves

Left AV (mitral) valve

Pulmonary valve

Aortic valve

Right AV (tricuspid) valve

Left ventricle

Right ventricle

A

S
L ↔ R
I

1

2

3

Skeleton of heart

4

5

6

B

C

A
L ↔ R
P

Ventricles relaxed

Ventricles contracted

(From Thibodeau GA, Patton KT: *Anatomy and physiology*, ed 6, St. Louis, 2007, Mosby.)

C, Principal arteries and veins.

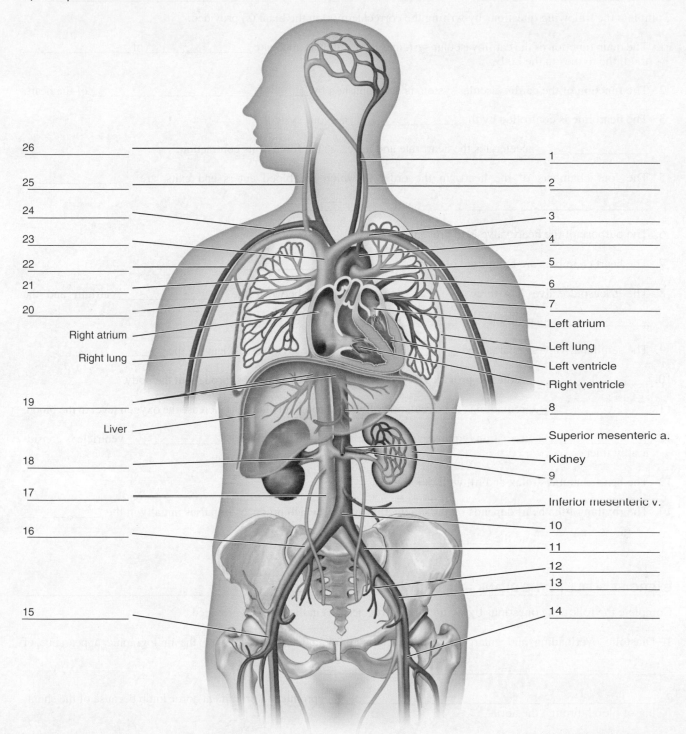

26 _____

25 _____

24 _____

23 _____

22 _____

21 _____

20 _____

Right atrium _____

Right lung _____

19 _____

Liver _____

18 _____

17 _____

16 _____

15 _____

1 _____

2 _____

3 _____

4 _____

5 _____

6 _____

7 _____

Left atrium

Left lung

Left ventricle

Right ventricle

8 _____

Superior mesenteric a.

Kidney

9 _____

Inferior mesenteric v.

10 _____

11 _____

12 _____

13 _____

14 _____

(From Solomon P, Solomon MK, Edelson-Solomon K: *Introduction to human anatomy and physiology*, ed 3, St. Louis, 2009, Saunders.)

EXERCISE 2: FILL IN THE BLANK—ANATOMY AND PHYSIOLOGY

Complete the following questions by writing the correct term(s) in the blank(s) provided.

1. The main function of the cardiovascular system is to maintain an adequate _____ of _____ to all the tissues in the body.

2. The function of the cardiovascular system is accomplished by _____ _____ of the heart.

3. The heart rate is controlled by the _____ nervous system.

4. _____ accelerates the heart rate and increases the force of its contraction.

5. The four chambers of the heart, in the order in which the blood enters and exits, are _____, _____, _____, and _____.

6. The purpose of the heart valve is to prevent _____.

7. The heart chambers are composed of _____ _____.

8. The tricuspid valve has three _____ and is between the _____ atrium and the _____ ventricle.

9. The semilunar valves separate the _____ from the great vessels leaving the _____.

10. _____ circulation provides oxygen and nourishment to tissues throughout the body.

11. _____ circulation is the circulation of blood through the lungs to increase the oxygen level in the blood.

12. _____ circulation requires a greater pressure so the wall of the _____ ventricle is considerably thicker.

13. The heart chambers relax and fill with blood during _____.

14. The rhythm of the heart depends on the conduction system, which produces impulses initially in the _____ _____ and the _____ _____.

EXERCISE 3: FILL IN THE BLANK—CARDIOVASCULAR PATHOLOGY

Complete the following questions by writing the correct term(s) in the blank(s) provided.

1. Diastolic overloading and enlargement of the left atrium and left ventricle are the radiographic appearance of _____ _____ _____.

2. _____ _____ _____ produces a prominent aortic knob because of the shunting of blood through the aorta.

3. Tetralogy of Fallot consists of a combination of the four abnormalities: _____, _____, _____, and _____.

4. _____ of the aorta causes a decreased blood flow to the abdomen and legs because of the constriction of the vessel.

5. In most patients, coronary artery narrowing is caused by deposits of _____ material on the inner arterial wall.

6. Death of the myocardium caused by coronary artery occlusion is referred to as a _____

   _____.

7. Fifty percent of coronary artery disease occurs in the _____ coronary artery.

8. In percutaneous transluminal coronary angioplasty, a balloon catheter is used to _____ the constricted coronary artery.

9. The four associated radiographic appearances related to left-sided heart failure are the _____,

   _____, _____, and _____.

10. The radiographer can influence the size of the heart on an image by changing the following three positioning criteria: _____, _____, and _____.

11. Cardiomegaly is evaluated using the _____ ratio.

12. The most common cause of pulmonary edema is elevated _____ _____ pressure.

13. A loss of normal sharp definition of the pulmonary vascular markings occurs in _____ _____.

14. Blood pressure depends on the following two factors: _____ and _____.

15. The two types of aneurysms are _____ and _____.

16. A kidney-ureter-bladder (KUB) radiograph demonstrates a curvilinear _____ in the wall of an aneurysm.

17. The danger of an aneurysm is its tendency to enlarge and rupture, leading to _____ _____, which may be fatal if it involves a critical organ such as the brain.

18. In cases of closed chest trauma, the imaging signs in addition to mediastinal widening that are important for a definitive diagnosis of rupture of the aorta are _____, _____, and _____.

19. An intravascular clot is called a(n) _____.

20. _____ is the most sensitive and most specific noninvasive method for diagnosing mitral stenosis.

EXERCISE 4: MATCHING—ANATOMY AND PHYSIOLOGY

Match each of the following terms with the correct definition by placing the letter of the best answer in the space provided. Each question has only one correct answer. Please note that there are more terms than definitions.

1. _____ chambers receiving blood from the great vessels

2. _____ band of atypical cardiac muscle fibers

3. _____ circulatory process of oxygenating the blood and removing waste products

4. _____ contraction phase of the heart

5. _____ double membranous sac surrounding the heart

6. _____ excitable components with the ability to create impulses

7. _____ four chambers composed of myocardium

8. _____ larger and thicker chambers providing circulation of the blood

9. _____ prevents backflow between the right atrium and right ventricle

10. _____ provides the body with blood

11. _____ separates the ventricles and the great vessels leaving the heart

12. _____ stimulates mechanical contraction of the atria

A. atria

B. atrioventricular (AV) node

C. conduction system

D. bundle of His

E. diastole

F. heart

G. intrinsic rhythm

H. mitral valve

I. pericardium

J. pulmonary circulation

K. semilunar valve

L. sinoatrial (SA) node

M. systemic circulation

N. systole

O. tricuspid valve

P. ventricles

EXERCISE 5: MATCHING—CARDIOVASCULAR PATHOLOGY

Match each of the following terms with the correct definition by placing the letter of the best answer in the space provided. Each question has only one correct answer. Please note that there are more terms than definitions.

1. _____ abnormal accumulation of fluid in the extravascular tissue

2. _____ accumulation of fluid within the space surrounding the heart

3. _____ closed-chest trauma with mediastinal widening

4. _____ develop in the veins where blood flow is static (or slow)

5. _____ diffuse thickening of the valve by fibrous tissue or calcific deposits

6. _____ dilated elongated tortuous vessels

7. _____ disruption of the inner layer of the blood vessel that allows blood to enter the wall of the aorta

8. _____ fatty material of the inner arterial wall

9. _____ free communication between the atria resulting from the lack of closure of the foramen ovale

10. _____ generalized tortuosity and elongation of the ascending aorta

11. _____ inability of the heart to provide the body with an adequate blood supply

12. _____ leading cause of strokes and congestive heart failure

13. _____ most common cause of cyanotic congenital heart disease

14. _____ narrowing of arteries causing oxygen deprivation of the myocardium

15. _____ narrowing or constriction of the aorta

16. _____ obstruction of the left ventricular outflow increases the workload of the left ventricle

17. _____ part or all of the clot becomes detached from the vessel wall

18. _____ saccular and fusiform are types

19. _____ symptom of hardened arteries that have a loss of elasticity

20. _____ vessel connecting the pulmonary artery and the aorta

A. aneurysm

B. aortic dissection

C. aortic rupture

D. aortic stenosis

E. atherosclerosis

F. atrial septal defect

G. coarctation of the aorta

H. congestive heart failure

I. coronary artery disease

J. embolism

K. hypertension

L. hypertensive heart disease

M. infective endocarditis

N. mitral insufficiency

O. mitral stenosis

P. patent ductus arteriosus

Q. pericardial effusion

R. plaque

S. pulmonary edema

T. rheumatic heart disease

U. tetralogy of Fallot

V. thrombosis

W. varicose veins

X. ventricular septal defect

Circle the best answer for each of the following multiple choice questions.

1. The most common congenital cardiac lesion is
   a. atrial septal defect
   b. patent ductus arteriosus
   c. ventricular septal defect
   d. tetralogy of Fallot

2. _____ is becoming the modality of choice to image congenital heart disease because both the morphologic and the functional anomalies can be visualized.
   a. Computed tomography (CT)
   b. Ultrasound (US)
   c. Magnetic resonance imaging (MRI)
   d. Nuclear medicine (NM)

3. The classic coeur en sabot appearance, in which the heart resembles the curved-toe portion of the wooden shoe, appears in cases of
   a. tetralogy of Fallot
   b. coarctation
   c. patent ductus arteriosus
   d. atrial septal defect

4. Coarctation of the aorta is demonstrated radiographically as
   a. rib notching and two bulges in the region of the aortic knob
   b. an enlarged heart
   c. an enlarged left atrium and ventricle
   d. coeur en sabot

5. The most commonly used noninvasive study to assess regional blood flow and tissue viability of the myocardium is
   a. CT
   b. MRI
   c. NM perfusion scan
   d. coronary arteriography

6. The definitive procedure to determine the presence and severity of coronary artery disease is
   a. CT
   b. computed radiography
   c. NM perfusion scan
   d. coronary arteriography

7. Right-sided heart failure causes
   a. a lack of blood flow to the organs
   b. a lack of blood flow into the systemic circulation
   c. a lack of blood flow to the extremities
   d. a backflow of blood in the venous systemic circulation

8. The butterfly or bat's-wing pattern, which is most prominent in the central portion of the lungs, is indicative of
   a. pulmonary effusion
   b. pulmonary edema
   c. congestive heart failure
   d. aortic coarctation

9. Of the following blood pressure values, which represents hypertension?
   a. 120/90
   b. 130/80
   c. 140/70
   d. 150/100

10. The string-of-beads pattern on a renal arteriogram suggests
    a. fibromuscular dysplasia
    b. emphysematous pyelonephritis
    c. atherosclerosis
    d. coarctation

11. A result of long-standing hypertension is
    a. atherosclerosis
    b. fibromuscular dysplasia
    c. hypertensive heart disease
    d. dilated arteries

12. Localized dilatation of an artery is a(n)
    a. aneurysm
    b. dissection
    c. rupture
    d. embolism

13. Which of the following is/are a type(s) of aneurysm?
    a. saccular
    b. fusiform
    c. weakness in the blood vessel wall
    d. all of the above

14. For abdominal aortic aneurysms, the noninvasive modality or procedure of choice for initial detection is
    a. arteriography
    b. CT
    c. MRI
    d. US

15. To best demonstrate the location and extent of an aneurysm, the diagnostician's choice in imaging is
    a. computed tomography angiography (CTA)
    b. magnetic resonance angiography (MRA)
    c. US
    d. either a or b

100

16. _____ begins with an intimal tear in the aorta.
    a. Dissection
    b. Traumatic rupture
    c. Aneurysm
    d. Atherosclerosis

17. The classic double-barrel aorta is indicative of
    a. aortic rupture
    b. hypertension
    c. aortic dissection
    d. atherosclerosis

18. Fatty deposits in the artery cause
    a. plaques
    b. hemorrhages
    c. ruptures
    d. tears

19. To demonstrate venous patency in varicose veins, the procedure of choice is
    a. CTA of the lower legs
    b. lower leg venography
    c. MRA of the lower extremities
    d. lower leg angiography

20. Bacteria or fungi from vegetations on the heart valves in
    a. infective carditis
    b. rheumatic heart disease
    c. mitral stenosis
    d. mitral insufficiency

EXERCISE 7: CASE STUDIES

The problems described in the following case studies required imaging related to the cardiovascular system. After each scenario, the images are presented, and you are asked to answer questions. Using your knowledge of imaging pathology, apply exposure factors and positioning criteria to answer the questions.

CASE STUDY 1

An adult male patient in the cardiac intensive care unit was experiencing SOB (shortness of breath).
A portable chest x-ray was ordered; the following image was obtained:

1. How was the patient positioned for this image?

What evidence is provided to indicate the patient position?

2. How does the positioning in this case influence heart size?

3. What other positioning factors could cause changes in the heart size?

4. What disease process may be misdiagnosed if the radiographer does not label the image properly?

5. How large should the heart appear on an image?

Does the heart appear to be of normal size and shape? Describe the changes, if any.

Why will the radiologist realize that the change in the position has occurred?

6. What ratio is used to determine whether the heart is enlarged?

The patient in this case has had a heart transplant. This image, if provided without a history, comparison images, or proper labeling, could be misdiagnosed. The image was compared with a previous image for the most accurate diagnosis. In this case, the image is considered normal for this patient. The shadow on the right, which seems to indicate an enlarged heart, is the patient's original heart.

CASE STUDY 2

A patient enters the CT department with an order for an abdominal scan to rule out abdominal aortic aneurysm; the following image was obtained:

1. The aorta is anatomically located anterior to the spine and normally appears as an oval area slightly to the left. In this instance, is the aorta seen as described?

Chapter **7** **Cardiovascular System**

2. There is a mass located anterior to the spine in which small white spots are embedded. What represents white on CT images and might be found in the walls of a blood vessel (the aorta)?

3. Could these deposits be seen on an abdominal image?

4. In image B, the diameter of the aorta demonstrates what abnormality, with a hematoma (on the left and posterior, seen with soft tissue attenuation but has a very ragged edge)?

5. The anatomic structures represent what region of the abdomen on image C?

6. What are the arteries in this area (image C)?

7. Do the same deposits appear? Where?

CT has the ability to identify the location and extent of an abdominal aortic aneurysm. The width of the abdominal aortic aneurysm in this case is 9 cm. Contrast material was not required, which gives CT an advantage over traditional angiography.

SELF-TEST

Read each question carefully, then circle the best answer.

1. Varicose veins usually involve the
    a. deep veins
    b. external arteries
    c. internal arteries
    d. superficial veins

2. DVT (deep venous thrombosis) can be caused by
    a. electrolyte imbalance
    b. oral contraceptives
    c. exercise
    d. diet

3. For diagnosing DVT with a noninvasive approach, the modality with 95% accuracy is
    a. CTA
    b. MRA
    c. duplex color Doppler US
    d. venography

4. On echocardiography, a posterior sonolucent fluid collection surrounding the heart is suggestive of
    a. pericardial effusion
    b. pleural edema
    c. pleural effusion
    d. pulmonary edema

5. The development of nodules or vegetations on the heart valves caused by bacteria or fungi is indicative of
    a. rheumatic fever
    b. pericarditis
    c. mitral stenosis
    d. infective carditis

6. _____ is a disorder that can be caused by syphilis, infective carditis, a dissection aneurysm, or Marfan syndrome.
    a. Aortic insufficiency
    b. Mitral insufficiency
    c. Mitral stenosis
    d. Rheumatic fever

7. Regurgitation indicates
    a. backflow of blood
    b. dilation of a blood vessel
    c. stenosis of a vessel
    d. that infection has inflamed a vessel

Chapter **7 Cardiovascular System**

8. Valve insufficiency occurs in patients with
   a. pericardial effusion
   b. rheumatic heart disease
   c. aneurysms
   d. poor cardiac output

9. A complication of infective carditis is
   a. mitral insufficiency
   b. pericardial effusion
   c. rheumatic heart disease
   d. septic emboli

10. The most common underlying disorder causing renovascular hypertension is
    a. fibromuscular dysplasia
    b. arteriosclerosis
    c. atherosclerosis
    d. aortic aneurysm

11. An aortic dissection is a
    a. hemorrhage into the mediastinum
    b. rupture of the aorta
    c. tear in the intima
    d. tear in the muscularis

12. A hemorrhage into the mediastinum causes a mediastinal widening and a loss of a discrete aortic knob shadow in
    a. dissection of the aorta
    b. traumatic aortic rupture
    c. abdominal aortic aneurysm
    d. hypertensive heart disease

13. To identify a clot within an aneurysm, the modality of choice is
    a. abdominal aortogram
    b. CTA
    c. Doppler US
    d. none of the above

14. A saccular aneurysm is defined as a(n)
    a. inward vascular growth
    b. enlarged vessel circumference
    c. outpouching only on one side of the artery
    d. fatty deposit

15. Fatty deposits in the artery cause
    a. plaques
    b. hemorrhages
    c. ruptures
    d. tears

16. A weakness in the wall of an artery causing a dilatation is evidence of a(n)
    a. plaque
    b. aneurysm
    c. dissection
    d. rupture

17. The continued strain of what condition leads to dilatation and enlargement of the left ventricle?
    a. hypertensive heart disease
    b. fibromuscular dysplasia
    c. dissection of the aorta
    d. pulmonary emboli

18. In hypertensive heart disease, the narrowing of the systemic circulation causes
    a. an aneurysm
    b. high blood pressure
    c. the left ventricle to assume an increased workload
    d. the right ventricle's workload to increase

19. _____ is most commonly seen in young women and appears radiographically as a string-of-beads pattern.
    a. Hypertension
    b. Fibrous dysplasia
    c. Hypertensive heart disease
    d. Atherosclerosis

20. Essential hypertension characterized by a gradual onset and a prolonged course is a
    a. secondary form
    b. malignant form
    c. idiopathic form
    d. benign form

21. _____ refers to an abnormal accumulation of fluid in the extravascular pulmonary tissue.
    a. Pulmonary emboli
    b. Pulmonary effusion
    c. Pulmonary edema
    d. Hypertensive heart disease

22. A bilateral symmetrical fan-shaped infiltration seen on a posteroanterior chest radiograph is the characteristic
    _____ sign of _____.
    a. butterfly; pulmonary edema
    b. string-of-beads; fibrous dysplasia
    c. coeur en sabot; hypertensive heart disease
    d. cobra; uterocele

23. The cardiothoracic (C/T) ratio is used to evaluate
    a. mediastinal shift
    b. heart size
    c. body rotation
    d. pulmonary edema

24. When the heart lacks the ability to adequately supply the body with blood, the patient has
    a. congestive heart failure
    b. pericardial effusion
    c. hypertensive heart disease
    d. increased cardiac output

25. When coronary vascularization is occluded, the area of the myocardium loses its blood supply, causing
    a. rheumatic heart disease
    b. myocardial infarction
    c. hypertensive heart disease
    d. congestive heart failure

26. A constriction of the aorta causing reduced blood flow to the abdominal organs and the lower extremities is called

_____ of the aorta.
   a. rupture
   b. dissection
   c. coarctation
   d. ductus arteriosus

27. Cyanotic congenital heart disease consists of four abnormalities: high ventricular septal defect, overriding of the aortic orifice above the ventricular defect, right ventricular hypertrophy, and
   a. mitral stenosis
   b. pulmonary stenosis
   c. tricuspid stenosis
   d. aortic stenosis

28. A vessel extending from the pulmonary artery to what vessel occurs in a patient with patent ductus arteriosus?
   a. aorta
   b. pulmonary vein
   c. superior vena cava
   d. left atrium

29. Free communication between the atria is _____, which has a left-to-right shunting effect.
   a. patent ductus arteriosus
   b. ventricular septal defect
   c. atrial septal defect
   d. tetralogy of Fallot

30. If the first impulse in the conduction system of the heart fails to fire, what structure will generate rhythmic impulses at a slower than normal rate?
   a. ectopic pacemaker
   b. sinoatrial node
   c. atrioventricular node
   d. bundle of His

8 Nervous System

OBJECTIVES

In addition to the objectives listed at the beginning of Chapter 8 in the textbook, the user should be able to:
1. Identify anatomic structures on diagrams and radiographs of the nervous system.
2. Describe the physiology of the nervous system.
3. Differentiate the pathologic disorders of the nervous system by defining the disease processes and their radiographic manifestations.
4. Determine changes in technical factors to obtain optimal-quality radiographs for patients with various underlying pathologic conditions.

EXERCISE 1: LABELING—ANATOMY

Identify the anatomic structures indicated by writing the correct names in the spaces provided.

A, Structure of a neuron.

(From Solomon P: *Introduction to human anatomy and physiology*, ed 4, St. Louis, 2016, Saunders.)

B, Divisions of the brain.

S
A ✦ P
I

1 _____
2 _____

11 _____
10 _____
9 _____
8 _____

7 _____
6 _____
5 _____
4 _____

3 _____

(From Vidic B, Suarez FR: *Photographic atlas of the human body*, St. Louis, 1984, Mosby.)

C, Covering structures of the central nervous system.

2 _____
1 _____
12 _____
3 _____
5 _____
6 _____
7 _____
4 _____
11 _____
10 _____
9 _____
8 _____

S
P ✦ A
I

S
R ✦ L
I

(From Thibodeau GA, Patton KT: *Anatomy and physiology*, ed 7, St. Louis, 2010, Mosby.)

EXERCISE 2: FILL IN THE BLANK—ANATOMY AND PHYSIOLOGY

Complete the following questions by writing the correct term(s) in the blank(s) provided.

1. The _____ _____ system consists of the cranial, spinal, and autonomic nerves.

2. _____ neurons, also known as sensory neurons, carry impulses to the central nervous system from the peripheral receptors.

3. Efferent neurons conduct impulses away from the _____ to the _____ _____.

4. The smooth muscle, cardiac muscle, and glandular epithelial tissue are controlled by the _____ nervous system.

5. The basic unit of the nervous system is the _____.

6. A single threadlike extension, a(n) _____, leads away from the nerve cell body.

7. To increase the rate of transmission of nervous impulses, the axon is insulated by the _____.

8. A chemical reaction permits the travel of impulses from the dendrite to the next axon at the _____.

9. The basic _____ _____ consists of an afferent, or sensory, neuron, which conducts impulses to the CNS from the periphery; and an efferent, or motor, neuron, which conducts impulses from the CNS to peripheral effectors.

10. The neurons that carry the impulse to the skeletal muscle to cause movement are called the _____ or _____ neurons.

11. The thin layer of gray matter where nerve cell bodies are concentrated is the _____ of the cerebrum.

12. The two hemispheres are called the _____.

13. High elevated convolutions on the surface of the cerebrum are the _____.

14. _____ matter is the inner area of the cerebrum consisting of nerve fiber tracts.

15. The cerebral cortex is responsible for receiving _____ information from the body and for triggering impulses to control _____ activity.

16. _____ impulses are transmitted to the posterior portion of the brain.

17. Stimulation on one side of the cerebral cortex causes contraction of muscle on the _____ side of the body.

18. The _____ _____ connects the two cerebral hemispheres by a mass of white matter.

19. The caudate nuclei, globus pallidus, and putamen make up the _____ _____.

20. The _____ is composed of the midbrain, the pons, and the medulla.

21. The coordination of muscle groups by the _____ helps maintain equilibrium and posture.

22. The outer protective covering of the brain is the _____.

23. The three meningeal layers, from the innermost to the outer layer, are the _____, _____, and _____.

24. The third and fourth ventricles are connected by the _____ of _____.

25. The superior portion of the third ventricle, which connects the lateral ventricles, is known as the _____ of _____.

26. The choroid plexus is located in the _____ ventricles and the roofs of the third and fourth ventricles.

27. The _____ _____ is a tentlike covering over the cerebellum that separates it from the occipital lobe of the cerebrum.

28. The _____ is a relay station that receives and processes sensory information.

29. The two divisions of the nervous system are the _____ and _____.

30. The three structures found in the diencephalon are the _____, _____, and _____.

EXERCISE 3: FILL IN THE BLANK—NERVOUS SYSTEM PATHOLOGY

Complete the following questions by writing the correct term(s) in the blank(s) provided.

1. Mumps, polio, and possibly herpes simplex cause _____ _____.

2. Acute inflammation of the meninges (pia mater and arachnoid) is _____.

3. Mild headaches and fever to more severe cerebral dysfunction, seizures, and a coma may result from the viral infection of the brain called _____.

4. The most common form of meningitis is caused by _____ _____, _____, and _____.

5. An area with poorly defined borders and a mass effect reflecting vascular congestion and edema represent the earliest signs of a(n) _____ _____ on computed tomography (CT) and magnetic resonance imaging (MRI).

6. _____ is the procedure of choice to demonstrate a crescentic or lentiform extraaxial fluid collection adjacent to the skull border as seen in a subdural empyema.

7. In _____ empyema, the infectious process is localized outside the dural membrane.

8. _____ _____ is a suppurative process in the space between the inner surface of the dura and the outer surface of the arachnoid.

9. A _____ fracture is a linear fracture that intersects a skull suture and courses along it.

10. A stellate fracture has multiple fracture lines radiating outward from a central point, is usually found in the skull, and is also known as a _____ fracture.

11. The three different types of cerebral hematomas are _____, _____, and _____.

12. An epidural hematoma appears as a _____ peripheral high-density lesion on a CT scan of the brain.

13. A(n) _____ hematoma demonstrates an increased density that has a crescentic shape adjacent to the inner table of the skull.

14. The frontal and anterior temporal regions are the most common sites of injury, demonstrating edema and hemorrhage, in cases of _____ _____.

15. Bleeding, which appears as increased density within the basilar cisterns, cerebral fissures, and sulci, indicates a(n) _____ _____.

16. The face consists of thin, poorly supported bones that easily _____ in response to a traumatic force.

17. The _____ fracture can be hammock-like or the trapdoor variety, which is best demonstrated on _____.

18. The submentovertex projection best demonstrates _____ _____ fractures.

19. A(n) _____ fracture results in a free-floating zygoma, causing disfiguration if not treated.

20. The angle of the _____ is the most common fracture site in the jaw.

21. The most common facial fracture is a fracture of the _____ _____.

22. Processes causing _____ _____ include abnormal vessel walls, occlusions, blood vessel ruptures, and decreased blood flow.

23. Imaging evaluation in acute strokes is performed to _____ or _____ other disorders that simulate the same clinical findings.

24. An embolic stroke or stenosis causing a temporary blockage of a cerebral vessel is a(n) _____.

25. A _____ scan is used as a screening study to demonstrate the carotid artery.

26. With a fresh bleed, the CT scan demonstrates a homogeneously dense, well-defined lesion with a round to oval configuration in cases of a(n) _____ hemorrhage.

EXERCISE 4: FILL IN THE BLANK—NERVOUS SYSTEM PATHOLOGY

Complete the following questions by writing the correct term(s) in the blank(s) provided.

1. _____ is the most sensitive technique for detecting most suspected brain tumors.

2. Seizure disorders and gradual neurologic deficits are the clinical signs of a _____ of the central nervous system.

3. A(n) _____ _____ usually originates in the internal auditory canal and extends into the cerebellopontine angle cistern.

4. A nonsecreting pituitary adenoma is called a _____ _____.

5. _____ have calcifications that usually can be detected on plain skull images.

6. Rapidly growing germ cell tumors occurring more frequently in males are the _____ and _____.

7. Ill-defined bone destruction or cortical expansion and a flocculent calcification are the radiographic appearances suggestive of a _____.

8. In MRI, single or multiple masses presenting high signal intensity on a T2-weighted image situated at the junction between gray matter and white matter is/are _____ _____.

9. _____ _____ is the mildest type of epilepsy, which occurs primarily in children.

10. _____ is the modality of choice to localize the seizure focus in a patient with hippocampal sclerosis.

11. Ventricular dilatation with prominent sulci in the cerebral hemispheres is indicative of _____ _____.

12. The four characteristics of Parkinson's disease are _____, _____, _____, and _____.

13. Atrophy of the caudate nucleus and putamen is the hallmark of _____ disease.

14. The two types of hydrocephalus are _____ and _____.

15. Mucosal thickening most commonly seen in the maxillary antra is _____.

EXERCISE 5: MATCHING—ANATOMY

Match each of the following terms with the correct definition by placing the letter of the best answer in the space provided. Each question has only one correct answer. Please note that there are more terms than definitions.

1. _____ afferent and efferent neurons

2. _____ fatty covering providing insulation

3. _____ impulse conducted to and from the CNS

4. _____ carries impulses away from the central nervous system to the peripheral effectors

5. _____ junction between neurons

6. _____ nerve cell

7. _____ one or more threadlike extensions leading toward a cell body

8. _____ supplies the striated skeletal muscles

9. _____ the brain and spinal cord

10. _____ conducts impulses from the peripheral receptors to the central nervous system

A. autonomic nervous system

B. axon

C. central nervous system

D. dendrite

E. motor neurons

F. myelin sheath

G. neuron

H. peripheral nervous system

I. reflex arc

J. sensory neurons

K. somatic nervous system

L. synapse

EXERCISE 6: MATCHING—NEUROANATOMY

Match each of the following terms with the correct definition by placing the letter of the best answer in the space provided. Each question has only one correct answer. Please note that there are more terms than definitions.

1. _____ absorbs cerebrospinal fluid into the venous blood circulation

2. _____ acts with the cerebral cortex to produce skilled movements by coordinating muscle groups

3. _____ houses cerebrospinal fluid

4. _____ connects the two cerebral hemispheres

5. _____ controls position and automatic movement

6. _____ convoluted elevations

7. _____ deep grooves dividing cerebral hemispheres

8. _____ delicate weblike middle covering of the central nervous system

9. _____ largest part of the brain

10. _____ link between the mind and body

11. _____ outer portion of the cerebrum

12. _____ produces cerebrospinal fluid

13. _____ resembles a worm coiled on itself

14. _____ separates the cerebral hemispheres

15. _____ shallow grooves

16. _____ superior portion of the brainstem

17. _____ three membranes providing protection for the central nervous system

18. _____ tough outer covering of the brain

A. aqueduct of Sylvius

B. arachnoid membrane

C. arachnoid villi

D. basal ganglia

E. cerebellum

F. cerebrum

G. choroid plexus

H. corpus callosum

I. cortex

J. diencephalon

K. dura mater

L. falx cerebelli

M. falx cerebri

N. fissures

O. foramen of Monro

P. hypothalamus

Q. gyri

R. medulla

S. meninges

T. midbrain

U. pia mater

V. pons

W. subarachnoid space

X. sulci

Y. thalamus

Z. vermis

Match each of the following terms with the correct definition by placing the letter of the best answer in the space provided. Each question has only one correct answer. Please note that there are more terms than definitions.

1. _____ acute arterial bleed commonly over the parietotemporal convexity

2. _____ almost invariably associated with osteomyelitis

3. _____ any process caused by an abnormality of the blood vessels or blood supply to the brain

4. _____ appears radiographically as multiple small, poorly defined areas of lucency

5. _____ bilateral and horizontal fracture of the maxillae

6. _____ commonly caused by *Haemophilus influenzae* in neonates and young adults

7. _____ direct blow to the front of the orbit caused by a rapid increase in intraorbital pressure

8. _____ focal neurologic deficit that completely resolves in 24 hours

9. _____ fractures of the zygomatic arch and orbital floor, and a separation of the zygomaticofrontal suture

10. _____ caused by hypertensive vascular disease

11. _____ injury to the surface veins, cerebral parenchyma, or cortical arteries, or rupture of an aneurysm

12. _____ loculated infection most often in the gray matter

13. _____ most commonly ruptured veins between the dura and the arachnoid

14. _____ occurs when the brain comes in contact with the rough skull surfaces

15. _____ penetrating trauma to the neck that possibly results in a traumatic fistula

16. _____ sharp lucent line

17. _____ shearing forces tearing the arteries

18. _____ sudden and dramatic development of a focal neurologic deficit

19. _____ suppurative process between the dura mater and arachnoid

20. _____ viral inflammation of the brain and meninges

A. abscess

B. bacterial meningitis

C. blowout fracture

D. carotid artery injury

E. cerebral contusion

F. cerebrovascular disease

G. encephalitis

H. epidural empyema

I. epidural hematoma

J. intracerebral hematoma

K. intraparenchymal hemorrhage

L. Le Fort fracture

M. osteomyelitis of the skull

N. sinusitis

O. skull fracture

P. stroke syndrome

Q. subarachnoid hemorrhage

R. subdural empyema

S. subdural hematoma

T. transient ischemic attack

U. tripod fracture

V. viral meningitis

Match each of the following terms with the correct definition by placing the letter of the best answer in the space provided. Each question has only one correct answer. Please note that there are more terms than definitions.

1. _____ abnormal cells reaching the brain by hematogenous spread

2. _____ arises from remnants of the embryonic neural tube, most often at the clivus or lower lumbosacral region

3. _____ benign tumor that has cystic and solid components and originates from embryonic remnants

4. _____ causes gigantism in adolescents and acromegaly in adults

5. _____ condition of the brain in which temporary disturbances occur, causing a range of signs

6. _____ dilatation of the ventricular system

7. _____ focal or generalized enlargement of cranial nerve VIII

8. _____ generalized convulsions associated with a fall, hypersalivation, and incontinence (bowel and bladder)

9. _____ germinomas and teratomas are types

10. _____ involuntary movements and early dementia

11. _____ most common primary malignant brain tumor consisting of glial cells

12. _____ normal aging, which results in enlargement of the ventricular system and sulci, causing forgetfulness

13. _____ progressive cerebral atrophy developing at an earlier age than the senile period

14. _____ shaking palsy with stooped posture, stiffness, and slow movement with a fixed facial expression

15. _____ slow-growing tumors that form large cavities or pseudocysts

16. _____ tumor arising from arachnoid lining cells and attached to the dura mater

17. _____ viral infection of upper respiratory tract

18. _____ widespread selective atrophy and loss of motor nerve cells leading to extensive paralysis

A. acoustic neuroma

B. Alzheimer's disease

C. amyotrophic lateral sclerosis

D. astrocytoma

E. cerebellar atrophy

F. chordoma

G. craniopharyngioma

H. dementia

I. epilepsy

J. glioma

K. grand mal seizures

L. Huntington's disease

M. hydrocephalus

N. meningioma

O. metastatic carcinoma

P. multiple sclerosis

Q. Parkinson's disease

R. pineal tumor

S. pituitary adenoma

T. sinusitis

Circle the best answer for each of the following multiple choice questions.

1. The most common form of inflammation of the pia mater and arachnoid is
   a. bacterial meningitis
   b. encephalitis
   c. viral meningitis
   d. a brain abscess

2. Which of the following is *not* a membrane covering the brain?
   a. dura mater
   b. pia mater
   c. arachnoid
   d. epidural

3. Brain metastases usually originate in the
   a. testicles and kidney
   b. lung and breast
   c. breast and cervix
   d. colon and lung

4. A hematoma that occurs after a blunt head injury causing venous bleeding is a(n)
   a. epidural hematoma
   b. subarachnoid bleed
   c. subdural hematoma
   d. cerebral contusion

5. Movement of the brain within the calvaria following blunt trauma to the skull sometimes results in a cerebral
   a. subdural hematoma
   b. epidural hematoma
   c. acute hematoma
   d. contusion

6. Which of the following is the most common cause of a brain abscess?
   a. streptococci
   b. *Haemophilus influenzae*
   c. herpes simplex
   d. sinus infection

7. Sinus radiographs should be taken using a _____ beam and with the patient in the _____ position.
   a. vertical; recumbent
   b. vertical; prone
   c. horizontal; erect
   d. vertical; erect

8. The process associated with osteomyelitis, which appears as a low-density, poorly defined area adjacent to the inner skull table on CT, is a case of
   a. brain abscess
   b. epidural empyema
   c. subarachnoid empyema
   d. subdural empyema

9. A(n) _____ consists of the multiplication of glial cells, which spread by direct extension.
   a. glioma
   b. meningioma
   c. acoustic neuroma
   d. pituitary adenoma

10. A(n) _____ grows slowly, arising from the Schwann cells on the eighth cranial nerve.
    a. pituitary adenoma
    b. chromophobe adenoma
    c. acoustic neuroma
    d. meningioma

11. A meningioma is a benign tumor arising from
    a. arachnoid lining cells and is attached to the dura
    b. glial cells spreading by direct extension
    c. anterior lobe of the pituitary gland
    d. embryonic remnants

12. An air-fluid level seen in the sphenoid sinus is indicative of what type of skull fracture?
    a. basilar
    b. tripod
    c. blowout
    d. nasal bone

13. Rapidly growing germ cell tumors known as _____ are best demonstrated on MR sagittal images.
    a. pituitary tumors
    b. chordomas
    c. pineal tumors
    d. acoustic tumors

14. Tumors arising from the embryonic neural tube commonly found at the clivus are considered
    a. meningiomas
    b. chordomas
    c. neuromas
    d. gliomas

15. Acute arterial bleeding most commonly caused by a laceration of the medial meningeal artery is a

    _____ hematoma.
    a. subarachnoid
    b. subdural
    c. epidural
    d. intracerebral

16. Le Fort fractures result in a(n)
    a. detached fragment that is unstable and altered
    b. bilateral injury at the angle
    c. zygoma detachment
    d. inferior orbital rim fracture

17. Hemorrhagic strokes are most commonly caused by
    a. a berry aneurysm
    b. hypertension
    c. carotid artery disease
    d. a and b

18. Widespread selective atrophy with loss of neuromotor function leading to paralysis is
    a. hydrocephalus
    b. Alzheimer's disease
    c. Parkinson's disease
    d. amyotrophic lateral sclerosis

19. Scattered plaques of demyelination on MR images are lesions of
    a. multiple sclerosis
    b. epilepsy
    c. Alzheimer's disease
    d. Huntington's disease

20. The essence of the condition seems to be an inadequate

    production of dopamine in cases of _____ disease.
    a. Huntington's
    b. Parkinson's
    c. Alzheimer's
    d. epileptic

EXERCISE 10: CASE STUDIES

The problems described in the following case studies required imaging related to the nervous system. After each scenario, the images are presented, and you will be asked to answer questions. Using your knowledge of imaging pathology, apply exposure factors and positioning criteria to answer the questions.

CASE STUDY 1

A 45-year-old patient has a clinical workup, which included a nuclear medicine lung scan. The scan result was positive, so chest images were ordered. The following posteroanterior chest image and apical lordotic projection were obtained:

1. On image A and B, describe the area where the irregular radiopaque lesion is seen.

2. The area of interest needs to be better demonstrated, so what imaging could be used?

3. Before computerized tomography, conventional tomography was used to better delineate an anatomic structure or region. The slice thickness for tomographic imaging is controlled by what two factors?

4. The patient was also experiencing headaches, so a cerebral angiogram was completed, as shown in image C. The arrows represent an encircling stain representative of a(n) what? (Hint: What pathology has an enhancing rim?)

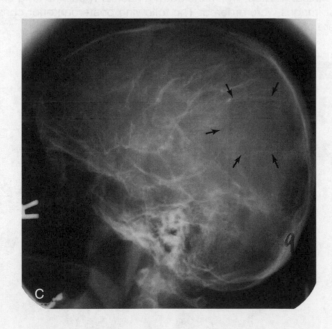

5. With the development of computerized technology, CT can demonstrate an abscess with better definition. On image A, the nonenhanced CT scan demonstrates a circular area with necrosis and possible liquefaction. On image B, the contrast-enhanced CT scan, what does the same area appear as?

CASE STUDY 2

A 71-year-old patient with a history of hypertension, chronic renal insufficiency, rheumatoid arthritis, and known carotid artery disease was evaluated. On physical examination, a bulging area on the neck was noticed, which also pulsated.

1. An angiogram was completed to study which artery?

2. When plaque disease (atherosclerosis) is demonstrated, the patient will go to surgery to have what procedure?

3. Following the surgery, the patient underwent color duplex Doppler ultrasound imaging to evaluate the carotid artery. The scan was abnormal, so a follow-up carotid arteriogram was performed. The following images demonstrate an outpouching, which is suggestive of what?

121

This patient's postoperative arteriogram was positive for a pseudoaneurysm. Doppler ultrasound imaging measured the pseudoaneurysm as 6 × 4 cm.

CASE STUDY 3

A young patient entered the emergency department with a severe headache. Skull radiographs demonstrated a mass of varying intensities caused by different blood flow rates in the region, as follows:

1. An irregular tangle of vessels and greatly dilated vessels is demonstrated on images A and B. What is this anatomic disorder known as?

2. In this case, neurointervention was accomplished. Compare image B with image C; why is the area of the malformation less visualized?

C

Detachable balloons were deployed to cause embolization. This saved the patient from undergoing surgery on the brain. There are still many risks involved with an interventional procedure, but the recovery period is much shorter.

A 1-month-old baby is brought to the radiology department for follow-up anteroposterior and lateral skull images, as shown here.

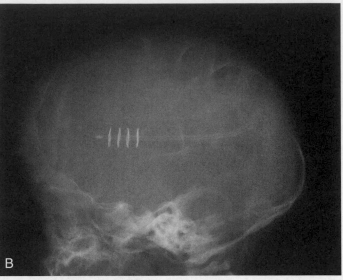

A   B

1. The inner table of the skull is uneven owing to increased internal fluid pressure. What is the name of the fluid?

2. What is the disorder of excessive fluid surrounding the brain tissue?

    What are the two types of this disorder?

3. On the image, there appears to be an artifact. What does this artifact represent? What is its purpose?

4. What imaging would best demonstrate the size of the fluid-filled spaces? Why?

This skull is said to have the lückenschädel appearance, which is caused by increased pressure from cerebrospinal fluid as a result of hydrocephalus.

SELF-TEST

Read each question carefully, then circle the best answer.

1. A viral inflammation of the brain and meninges is called
   a. meningitis
   b. hydrocephalus
   c. encephalitis
   d. encephalomalacia

2. The _____ space contains spinal fluid.
   a. subarachnoid
   b. epidural
   c. subdural
   d. epidermis

3. The imaging modality of choice to evaluate patients with suspected neurologic dysfunction caused by head trauma is
   a. ultrasound
   b. MRI
   c. CT
   d. skull radiography

4. A suppurative process in the space between the inner surface of the dura and the outer arachnoid surface is a(n)
   a. subdural empyema
   b. epidural empyema
   c. subarachnoid empyema
   d. brain abscess

5. A primary malignant tumor presenting high signal intensity on T2-weighted MR images is a(n)
   a. chromophobe adenoma
   b. acoustic neuroma
   c. glioma
   d. pituitary adenoma

6. A(n) _____ hematoma appears as a biconvex peripheral high-density lesion on CT.
   a. subdural
   b. epidural
   c. meningeal
   d. subarachnoid

7. Most _____ have calcifications, which can be visualized on routine skull images.
   a. meningiomas
   b. craniopharyngiomas
   c. gliomas
   d. chromophobe adenomas

8. A linear skull fracture that intersects the sutures and continues along the sutures is a _____ fracture.
   a. diastatic
   b. tripod
   c. zygomatic
   d. blowout

9. Bleeding into the ventricular system as a result of injury to the surface veins is a(n) _____ hemorrhage.
   a. intracerebral
   b. subarachnoid
   c. intraparenchymal
   d. subdural

10. _____ refers to any process caused by an abnormality of the blood supply to the brain.
    a. Cerebrovascular accident
    b. Cerebrovascular disease
    c. Stroke syndrome
    d. Transient ischemic attack

11. A disease process seen as scattered plaques on MR images as a result of demyelination is
    a. Parkinson's disease
    b. multiple sclerosis
    c. Huntington's disease
    d. amyotrophic lateral sclerosis

12. Atrophy of the caudate nucleus and putamen seen on CT as focal dilatation of the frontal horns with a loss of their normal shape is indicative of
    a. amyotrophic lateral sclerosis
    b. Huntington's disease
    c. multiple sclerosis
    d. Parkinson's disease

13. The tumor that grows slowly, has an infiltrating character, and can form large cavities and pseudocysts is a(n)
    a. meningioma
    b. chordoma
    c. acoustic neuroma
    d. astrocytoma

14. The rim of low intensity consisting of a cerebrospinal fluid cleft, the vascular rim, or dura demonstrating separation of the tumor from adjacent brain, seen on T1- and T2-weighted MR images, is
    a. meningioma
    b. chordoma
    c. acoustic neuroma
    d. astrocytoma

15. A fracture of the zygomatic arch and the orbital floor and a separation of the zygomaticofrontal suture is a _____ fracture.
    a. Le Fort
    b. tripod
    c. blowout
    d. linear

16. A loculated infection most commonly seen in the gray matter is
    a. a brain abscess
    b. bacterial meningitis
    c. a subdural empyema
    d. encephalitis

17. Increased intracranial pressure caused by a blockage is suggestive of
    a. normal-pressure hydrocephalus
    b. a grand mal seizure
    c. epilepsy
    d. noncommunicating hydrocephalus

18. A generalized convulsion that is associated with a fall, hypersalivation, and incontinence is considered
    a. epilepsy
    b. a grand mal seizure
    c. a petit mal seizure
    d. Parkinson's disease

19. Presenile progressive cerebral atrophy is also called _____ disease.
    a. Huntington's
    b. Lou Gehrig's
    c. Alzheimer's
    d. cerebrovascular

20. A berry aneurysm rupture is the major cause of a(n) _____ hemorrhage.
    a. intracerebral
    b. subdural
    c. epidural
    d. subarachnoid

Hematopoietic System

OBJECTIVES

In addition to the objectives listed at the beginning of Chapter 9 in the textbook, the user should be able to:
1. Identify anatomic structures on diagrams and radiographs of the hematopoietic system.
2. Describe the physiology of the hematopoietic system.
3. Differentiate the pathologic disorders of the hematopoietic system by defining the disease processes and their radiographic manifestations.
4. Determine changes in technical factors to obtain optimal-quality radiographs for patients with various underlying pathologic conditions.

EXERCISE 1: LABELING

Identify the anatomic structures indicated by writing the correct names in the spaces provided.

The formed elements of blood.

1 _____   2 _____

3 _____

4 _____

5 _____   6 _____   7 _____

8 _____

9 _____   10 _____

(From Thibodeau GA, Patton KT: *Anatomy and physiology*, ed 6, St. Louis, 2007, Mosby.)

EXERCISE 2: FILL IN THE BLANK—ANATOMY AND PHYSIOLOGY

Complete the following questions by writing the correct term(s) in the blank(s) provided.

1. Adequate blood supply brings the following four necessary components to the cells:

   _____, _____, _____, and _____.

2. Blood also provides a major defense system against _____, _____,

   and _____.

3. Blood-forming tissues in the body are _____ and _____.

4. Red bone marrow makes the following blood cells: _____, _____, and _____.

5. White blood cells are produced in the _____ and _____.

6. Name the five types of leukocytes:

   (i) _____

   (ii) _____

   (iii) _____

   (iv) _____

   (v) _____

7. The _____ defends the body against bacteria by ingesting the foreign microorganisms and destroying them.

8. The smallest blood cell provides the essentials for blood clotting and is the _____.

EXERCISE 3: FILL IN THE BLANK—HEMATOPOIETIC PATHOLOGY

Complete the following questions by writing the correct term(s) in the blank(s) provided.

1. A decreased amount of oxygen-carrying hemoglobin is present in the peripheral blood as a result of _____.

2. Three types of hemolytic anemia are _____, _____, and _____.

3. The fish vertebrae appearance occurs in _____ anemia and is caused by indentations on the superior and inferior margins of soft vertebral bodies.

4. The hair-on-end appearance consists of vertical striations in a radial pattern resulting from _____.

5. _____ anemia is caused by a lack of vitamin B12, or folic acid.

6. Severe chronic pulmonary disease or congenital cyanotic heart disease causes long-term inadequate oxygen supply in

   patients with _____ _____.

7. Because of cancer of the bone marrow, there is a huge increase in the number of circulating granulocytes and a

   decreased production of red blood cells and platelets in _____ _____.

8. A lymph node malignancy with a dramatic increase in lymphocytes is _____ _____.

9. As the disease progresses, bone destruction causing patchy lytic (moth-eaten) lesions may appear radiographically in cases of _____.

10. Neoplasms of the lymphoreticular system are _____.

11. The lymphoreticular system includes _____, _____, and _____.

12. Ninety percent of all lymphoma cases are _____ _____.

13. Hodgkin's lymphoma originates in _____ _____ in most cases.

14. Parenchymal organs are the originating point for _____ _____.

15. The most common radiographic finding in lymphoma is lymph node enlargement in the _____, which is bilateral but asymmetrical.

16. In lymphoma staging, _____ imaging can detect microscopic foci and function alterations in normal-size nodes.

17. Epstein-Barr virus may cause _____.

18. The three components required for coagulation to occur are _____, _____, and _____.

19. _____ causes hemorrhages in the small bowel, producing a characteristic uniform thickening of mucosal folds in the bowel segment affected.

EXERCISE 4: MATCHING—ANATOMY AND PHYSIOLOGY

Match each of the following terms with the correct definition by placing the letter of the best answer in the space provided. Each question has only one correct answer. Please note that there are more terms than definitions.

1. _____ an iron-based protein that carries the oxygen from the lungs to the cells in the body

2. _____ biconcave disks without nuclei that contain hemoglobin

3. _____ cell that plays a major role in the immune system and aids in the synthesis of antibodies

4. _____ contains granules that stain blue

5. _____ defends the body against bacteria

6. _____ red-staining cells that increase greatly in instances of allergy or parasitic conditions

7. _____ smallest blood cell, essential for clotting

8. _____ supplies nutrients, oxygen, salt, and hormones to the cells and carries away waste products

A. basophil

B. blood

C. coagulation factors

D. eosinophil

E. erythrocytes (red)

F. hemoglobin

G. leukocytes

H. lymphocytes

I. monocytes

J. neutrophil

K. platelets

Match each of the following terms with the correct definition by placing the letter of the best answer in the space provided. Each question has only one correct answer. Please note that there are more terms than definitions.

1. _____ anomaly of blood coagulation

2. _____ erythrocytes have an abnormal circular shape, making them vulnerable and susceptible to rupture

3. _____ generalized failure of the bone marrow function

4. _____ Hodgkin's and non-Hodgkin's

5. _____ hyperplasia of the bone marrow resulting in an increased production of red blood cells, granulocytes, and platelets

6. _____ neoplastic proliferation of white blood cells

7. _____ affected person appears pale because of a lack of hemoglobin in the blood

8. _____ radiographically seen as a tubular bald stomach, reflecting a decrease or absence of the usual rugal folds

9. _____ red blood cells are crescentic or sickle shaped and tend to rupture

10. _____ self-limited viral disease of the lymphoreticular system characterized by vague symptoms

11. _____ shortened red blood cell life span resulting in hemolysis

12. _____ spontaneous hemorrhages in the skin due to a deficiency in the number of platelets

A. anemia

B. aplastic anemia

C. hemolytic anemia

D. hemophilia

E. infectious mononucleosis

F. leukemia

G. lymphoma

H. megaloblastic anemia

I. myelocytic leukemia

J. pernicious anemia

K. polycythemia (primary)

L. purpura

M. sickle cell anemia

N. spherocytosis

O. thalassemia

EXERCISE 6: MULTIPLE CHOICE

Circle the best answer for each of the following multiple choice questions.

1. A decrease in the amount of oxygen-carrying hemoglobin in the peripheral blood is
   a. polycythemia
   b. leukemia
   c. anemia
   d. lymphoma

2. Spherocytosis, sickle cell anemia, and thalassemia are examples of what type of anemia?
   a. iron deficiency
   b. hemolytic
   c. pernicious
   d. myelophthisic

3. A defect in hemoglobin formation that occurs predominantly in persons living near the Mediterranean Sea is
   a. thalassemia
   b. megaloblastic anemia
   c. sickle cell anemia
   d. iron deficiency anemia

4. Gastric atrophy is seen radiographically as a tubular stomach with a bald appearance reflecting a decrease or absence of the usually prominent rugal folds indicates
   a. megaloblastic anemia
   b. sickle cell anemia
   c. polycythemia
   d. thalassemia

5. In sickle cell anemia, the red blood cells are
   a. crescent shaped
   b. circular and fragile
   c. biconcave
   d. not carrying oxygen

6. Aplastic anemia results in
   a. vitamin B12 deficiency
   b. decreased levels of erythrocytes and platelets
   c. decreased red and white blood cells
   d. hyperplasia of the bone marrow

7. Cancer of the bone marrow causing proliferation of white blood cells is
   a. lymphatic leukemia
   b. lymphoma
   c. polycythemia
   d. myelocytic leukemia

8. The most common radiographic finding in lymphoma is
   a. mediastinal lymph node enlargement
   b. splenomegaly
   c. prominent pulmonary vascular shadows
   d. localized steplike central depressions of the vertebrae

9. In cases of lymphoma, the best modality to demonstrate microscopic tumor foci is
   a. computed tomography (CT)
   b. magnetic resonance imaging (MRI)
   c. nuclear medicine
   d. positron emission tomography (PET)

10. A lifelong tendency for spontaneous hemorrhage is called
    a. hemolytic anemia
    b. mononucleosis
    c. hemophilia
    d. purpura

EXERCISE 7: CASE STUDY

In the following case study, pelvic imaging was requested. In this scenario you will see the images and will be asked to answer questions. Using your knowledge of imaging pathology, apply exposure factors and positioning criteria to answer the questions.

CASE STUDY 1

A man was previously diagnosed with Hodgkin's lymphoma. The patient underwent therapy and had been doing well. Currently the patient is experiencing middle and lower abdominal pain, so follow-up scans of the abdomen and pelvis were ordered, as shown:

The conglomerate lymph nodal mass is displacing the renal vein anteriorly, as demonstrated in image A.

Chapter **9** **Hematopoietic System**

1. Differentiate Hodgkin's and non-Hodgkin's lymphoma.

2. Which modalities are most useful in staging and treatment follow-up?

1: distance 104mm, angle 17
2: distance 89mm, angle 66

B

1: m 60.06,sd 11.27,a 179.49mm2
2: m 85.49,sd 15.09,a 32.31mm2
3: m -101.23,sd 13.78,a 32.31mm2

C

3. Referring to image B, what is the size of the mass (measurement)?

4. Three regions of interest (ROIs) were recorded on image C. What CT numbers are derived?

5. In which ROI is the CT number closest to the value of water?

6. Fat has a CT number less than 0. Which ROI would this be?

Read each question carefully, then circle the best answer.

1. When diseases of the hematopoietic system result in demineralization of bone, the radiographer must be alert to
   a. patient infection
   b. pathologic fracture
   c. self-infection
   d. parasites

2. White blood cells
   a. are the smallest blood cell and are required for clotting
   b. aid in the immune system and antibody synthesis
   c. carry hemoglobin
   d. are an iron-based protein that carries oxygen

3. Which term refers to a decrease in the amount of oxygen-carrying hemoglobin in the blood?
   a. thalassemia
   b. erythrocytosis
   c. anemia
   d. thrombocytopenia

4. Erythrocytes have an abnormal circular shape, which makes them vulnerable and susceptible to rupture in cases of
   a. thalassemia
   b. megaloblastic anemia
   c. thrombocytopenia
   d. spherocytosis

5. Thalassemia manifests radiographically as
   a. "hair-on-end" appearance of vertical striations in a radial pattern
   b. localized steplike central depressions of the vertebrae
   c. cardiomegaly
   d. gastric atrophy

6. Spontaneous hemorrhages in the skin caused by a lack of platelets is called
   a. hemophilia
   b. infectious mononucleosis
   c. purpura
   d. polycythemia

7. The anemia most often seen in African Americans, in which red cells are crescentic and tend to rupture, is
   a. sickle cell anemia
   b. thalassemia
   c. lymphoma
   d. thrombocytopenia

8. Abnormalities in blood coagulation are known as
   a. hemophilia
   b. aplastic anemia
   c. thrombocytopenia
   d. purpura

9. Aplastic anemia is associated with
   a. folic acid deficiency, causing loss of DNA synthesis
   b. generalized bone marrow failure
   c. proliferation of white blood cells
   d. neoplastic growths of the lymphoreticular system

10. The shortened life span of red blood cells is characteristic of what type of anemia?
    a. hemolytic
    b. iron deficiency
    c. megaloblastic
    d. pernicious

10 Endocrine System

OBJECTIVES

In addition to the objectives listed at the beginning of Chapter 10 in the textbook, the user should be able to:
1. Identify anatomic structures on diagrams and radiographs of the endocrine system.
2. Describe the physiology of the endocrine system.
3. Differentiate the pathologic disorders of the endocrine system by defining the disease processes and their radiographic manifestations.
4. Determine changes in technical factors to obtain optimal-quality radiographs for patients with various underlying pathologic conditions.

EXERCISE 1: LABELING—ANATOMY

Identify the anatomic structures indicated by writing the correct names in the spaces provided.

A, Adrenal gland.

1. _____
2. _____
3. _____
4. _____
5. _____

(From Thibodeau GA, Patton KT: *Anatomy and physiology*, ed 6, St. Louis, 2007, Mosby.)

B, Pituitary and hormones.

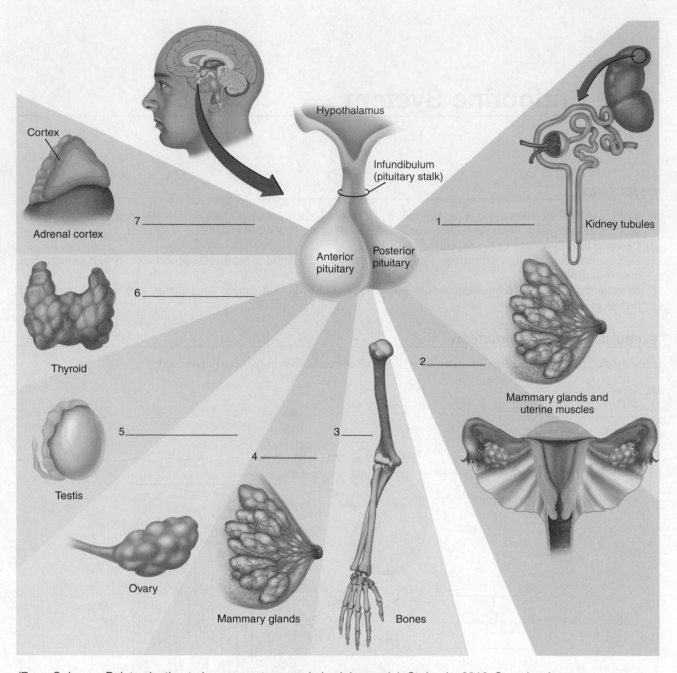

Hypothalamus

Infundibulum
(pituitary stalk)

Cortex

Adrenal cortex

Anterior
pituitary

Posterior
pituitary

Kidney tubules

7 _____

1 _____

Thyroid

6 _____

Mammary glands and
uterine muscles

2 _____

Testis

5 _____

3 _____

4 _____

Ovary

Mammary glands

Bones

(From Solomon P: *Introduction to human anatomy and physiology*, ed 4, St. Louis, 2016, Saunders.)

C, Thyroid and parathyroid glands.

1 _____

2 _____

3 _____

4 _____

5 _____

6 _____

7 _____

A

B

S
R ✛ L
I

(From Thibodeau GA, Patton KT: *Anatomy and Physiology*, ed 6, St. Louis, 2007, Mosby.)

EXERCISE 2: FILL IN THE BLANK—ANATOMY AND PHYSIOLOGY

Complete the following questions by writing the correct term(s) in the blank(s) provided.

1. The _____ _____ is situated on top of the kidney, and each component secretes different hormones.

2. _____ regulate salt and water balance by controlling kidney excretion of potassium and retention of sodium.

3. Glucocorticoids regulate _____ _____.

4. Androgens are sex hormones that _____, _____, and _____.

5. The adrenal medulla secretes _____ and _____, which are fight-or-flight hormones secreted in stressful situations when additional energy and strength are needed.

6. The hormonal secretions of the pituitary gland are controlled by the _____.

7. The pituitary gland sits in the bony depression in the spheroid bone called the _____ _____.

8. Growth hormone (GH) promotes _____ growth and _____ of the tissues.

9. Oxytocin is secreted by the _____ pituitary gland and causes contraction of _____ _____.

10. In response to the body's need for increased energy production, _____ stimulates cellular metabolism, which consists of iodine-containing substances.

11. The _____ _____ is a butterfly-shaped gland consisting of two lobes.

12. The _____ _____ are the glands responsible for controlling levels of blood calcium and phosphate.

13. Parathormone raises a low calcium level by the following three mechanisms: _____, _____, and _____.

14. _____ _____ is an endocrine disorder that commonly occurs when beta cells in the islets of Langerhans fail to secrete insulin.

EXERCISE 3: FILL IN THE BLANK—ENDOCRINE SYSTEM PATHOLOGY

Complete the following questions by writing the correct term(s) in the blank(s) provided.

1. Non-pituitary tumors producing ACTH may cause adrenal hyperfunction and _____ _____.

2. The most superficial layer of the adrenal cortex causes retention of sodium and water and an abnormal loss of potassium in the urine in cases of _____.

3. Elevated levels of androgens cause accelerated skeletal maturation along with premature epiphyseal fusion in _____ syndrome.

4. A typical higher signal intensity is seen on T2-weighted images in _____ metastasis demonstrating contrast enhancement.

5. Pheochromocytomas can be diagnosed with _____ _____; imaging only aids in confirmation.

6. About 50% of these tumors have calcifications, which distinguish them from Wilms' tumor; these calcifications represent _____.

7. Gigantism and acromegaly are examples of _____.

8. An excessively large skeleton is a manifestation of _____.

9. _____ causes profound generalized disturbances in bone growth and maturation.

10. Severe polyuria leads to massive dilatation of the renal pelves, calyces, and ureters in _____ _____.

11. The modality of choice to determine the function of the thyroid for both palpable and nonpalpable nodules is _____ _____.

12. A solid mass with a consistent echogenicity, often demonstrating a thick smooth periphery of a capsule, is a _____ _____ _____.

13. Name three types of thyroid carcinoma: _____, _____, and _____.

14. Name the three categories of hyperparathyroidism: _____, _____, and _____.

15. _____ _____ produces a variety of radiographic findings involving multiple systems, including atherosclerosis, susceptibility to infection, and neuropathy.

EXERCISE 4: MATCHING—ANATOMY AND PHYSIOLOGY

Match each of the following terms with the correct definition by placing the letter of the best answer in the space provided. Each question has only one correct answer. Please note that there are more terms than definitions.

1. _____ butterfly-shaped gland located in the neck

2. _____ control sodium retention and potassium secretion

3. _____ four tiny glands on the superior and inferior posterior aspects of the thyroid gland

4. _____ increases rate of absorption of water and electrolytes by the renal tubules

5. _____ inner medulla and outer cortex

6. _____ natural iodine-containing substance to stimulate cellular metabolism

7. _____ produces two hormones: vasopressin and oxytocin

8. _____ promotes growth and development of all parts of the body

9. _____ regulates carbohydrate metabolism

10. _____ regulates the menstrual cycle and the secretion of sex hormones (male and female)

11. _____ responsible for controlling calcium and phosphate blood levels

12. _____ secretes a group of hormones affecting the sex organs, or gonads

13. _____ sex hormones

14. _____ stimulates heart activity and raises blood pressure

15. _____ the master gland controlled by the hypothalamus

A. adrenal glands

B. androgens

C. anterior lobe of the pituitary gland

D. epinephrine

E. glucocorticoids

F. gonadotropin

G. growth hormone

H. hyperactive endocrine glands

I. luteinizing hormone

J. mineralocorticoids

K. oxytocin

L. parathormone

M. parathyroid glands

N. pituitary gland

O. posterior lobe of the pituitary gland

P. thyroid gland

Q. thyroxine

R. vasopressin (ADH)

141

Match each of the following terms with the correct definition by placing the letter of the best answer in the space provided. Each question has only one correct answer. Please note that there are more terms than definitions.

1. _____ a lack of insulin preventing glucose from entering cells

2. _____ characteristic obesity of the body's trunk and a moon-shaped face

3. _____ caused by overproduction of hormones; hypertension, muscular weakness, and excessive thirst are the results

4. _____ encapsulated mass usually compressing adjacent tissue

5. _____ enlargement of the thyroid gland not causing inflammation or neoplasia

6. _____ excessive growth hormone produced by a tumor

7. _____ excessive production of thyroxine

8. _____ exists in the adrenal medulla and produces excess vasopressors

9. _____ failure of normal end-organ response to normal levels of circulating hormones

10. _____ functional abnormality leading to an insufficient synthesis of thyroid hormone

11. _____ generalized disorder of calcium, phosphate, and bone metabolism

12. _____ kidneys' inability to conserve water, resulting in low blood levels of ADH (antidiuretic hormone)

13. _____ loss of secretion of any anterior pituitary hormone

14. _____ site to which pulmonary, breast, renal, and ovarian carcinomas most frequently spread

15. _____ most cases are caused by adrenocortical tumors

16. _____ papillary, follicular, and medullary are types of this neoplasia

17. _____ predominantly affects females symptomatically as nervousness, emotional liability, and inability to sleep

18. _____ rapidly growing mass usually necrotic at the time of clinical presentation

19. _____ symptoms are fatigue, anorexia, weakness, weight loss, hypotension, vomiting, and diarrhea

20. _____ ultrasound is the modality of choice to evaluate this abdominal mass in children

A. acromegaly

B. adrenal carcinoma

C. adrenal metastases

D. adrenogenital syndrome

E. aldosteronism

F. benign thyroid adenoma

G. Cushing's syndrome

H. diabetes insipidus

I. diabetes mellitus

J. goiter

K. Graves' disease

L. hyperglycemia

M. hyperparathyroidism

N. hyperpituitarism

O. hyperthyroidism

P. hypoadrenalism

Q. hypoparathyroidism

R. hypopituitarism

S. hypothyroidism

T. neuroblastoma

U. pheochromocytoma

V. pseudohypoparathyroidism

W. thyroid carcinoma

Circle the best answer for each of the following multiple choice questions.

1. Because of the radiographic changes produced in multiple systems, computed tomography (CT) is the modality of choice to evaluate for what disorder?
   a. aldosteronism
   b. adrenogenital syndrome
   c. Cushing's syndrome
   d. hypoadrenalism

2. In cases of what disorder is it the role of imaging to demonstrate the location of the adenoma, which will be difficult to detect during surgery?
   a. aldosteronism
   b. hypoadrenalism
   c. adrenal virilism
   d. Addison's disease

3. Excessive administration of steroids is the most common cause of
   a. aldosteronism
   b. hyperadrenalism
   c. adrenogenital syndrome
   d. hypoadrenalism

4. Adrenal carcinoma is best demonstrated on
   a. CT as a large irregular-edged mass
   b. US as a complex mass that is difficult to separate from the kidney
   c. magnetic resonance imaging (MRI) as an inflammatory process causing enlargement
   d. general radiography, a kidney-ureter-bladder (KUB) image

5. Arterial injections of iodinated contrast agents cause a sharp elevation in blood pressure in patients with
   a. neuroblastoma
   b. pheochromocytoma
   c. adrenal carcinoma
   d. adrenal metastasis

6. Thickened bones of the skull, enlarged paranasal sinuses, and lengthened mandible are all suggestive of
   a. hypopituitarism
   b. acromegaly
   c. hyperpituitarism
   d. hyperthyroidism

7. Which gland controls the level of secretion of gonadal and thyroid hormones and the production of GH?
   a. adrenal
   b. pituitary
   c. thyroid
   d. parathyroid

8. MRI is the modality of choice to demonstrate a pituitary tumor because of the
   a. multiplanar imaging abilities
   b. tumor size
   c. tumor location
   d. all of the above

9. Uniform radioactivity throughout a thyroid gland that demonstrates diffuse enlargement is suggestive of
   a. Addison's disease
   b. Graves' disease
   c. Conn's syndrome
   d. Cushing's syndrome

10. In severe cases of Graves' disease, the patient may have associated
    a. skeletal overgrowth and bone spurs
    b. generalized cardiomegaly and pulmonary congestion
    c. complex masses with an irregular periphery
    d. none of the above

11. An enlargement of the thyroid gland that is not inflammatory or neoplastic is
    a. a goiter
    b. an adenoma
    c. Graves' disease
    d. Addison's disease

12. The most common type of thyroid carcinoma is
    a. papillary
    b. medullary
    c. follicular
    d. cortical

13. Which of the following tumors spreads to regional lymph nodes and is slow growing and cystic?
    a. medullary carcinoma
    b. papillary carcinoma
    c. neuroblastoma
    d. pheochromocytoma

14. The thyroid carcinoma that closely mimics normal thyroid tissue is which type?
    a. follicular
    b. adenomatous
    c. medullary
    d. stem cell

15. Common manifestations of diabetes mellitus are
    a. polyuria, dysphagia, and hyperglycemia
    b. hyperglycemia, adenopathy, and polydipsia
    c. polyuria, polydipsia, and glycosuria
    d. hypoglycemic shock, polydipsia, and glycosuria

Read each question carefully, then circle the best answer.

1. The endocrine system controls
   a. a broad range of vital body activities
   b. a communication network through several glands
   c. secretion of chemical messengers
   d. all of the above

2. The hormones regulating carbohydrate metabolism are
   a. glucocorticoids
   b. androgens
   c. mineralocorticoids
   d. gonadotropins

3. Generalized enlargement of the adrenal glands is best demonstrated by
   a. ultrasound, appearing anechoic
   b. CT, appearing as thickened wings
   c. MRI, appearing as a functioning microadenoma
   d. none of the above

4. An abnormal loss of potassium in the urine can be caused by a(n)
   a. overproduction of mineralocorticoid hormones
   b. excessive amount of androgens
   c. abundance of glucocorticoids
   d. loss of androgens

5. Production of excessive androgenic active hormones by the adrenal gland causes
   a. Addison's disease
   b. Graves' disease
   c. Conn's syndrome
   d. adrenogenital syndrome

6. The most common cause of hypoadrenalism is
   a. steroid administration
   b. excessive mineralocorticoids
   c. excessive glucose
   d. excessive insulin

7. Because of rapid growth (usually necrotic), lymphatic and hepatic metastases are common when _____ manifests clinically.
   a. adrenal carcinoma
   b. neuroblastoma
   c. pheochromocytoma
   d. thyroid carcinoma

8. The carcinomas that most commonly metastasize to the adrenal gland are
   a. lung and prostate cancers
   b. breast and prostate cancers
   c. lung and breast cancers
   d. lung and brain cancers

9. The tumor that produces an excessive amount of vasopressor substances is a(n)
   a. adrenal carcinoma
   b. pheochromocytoma
   c. neuroblastoma
   d. aldosteronism

10. Calcifications have a fine granular or stippled appearance in
    a. pheochromocytoma
    b. neuroblastoma
    c. adrenal metastases
    d. thyroid goiter

11. The modality of choice to diagnose a neuroblastoma is
    a. CT
    b. ultrasound
    c. MRI
    d. nuclear medicine

12. The posterior lobe of the pituitary gland produces
    a. vasopressin and epinephrine
    b. oxytocin and norepinephrine
    c. vasopressin and oxytocin
    d. epinephrine and norepinephrine

13. Hyperpituitarism after bone growth has stopped causes
    a. gigantism
    b. elephantiasis
    c. acromegaly
    d. edema

14. Radiographers must be cautious of complications of Cushing's syndrome, such as
    a. sella erosion
    b. hypercalciuria
    c. spontaneous fractures
    d. frequent infections

15. The fight-or-flight hormones are
    a. androgen and adrenaline
    b. epinephrine and adrenaline
    c. glucocorticoid and androgen
    d. epinephrine and norepinephrine

16. The modality that demonstrates function of the thyroid gland the best is
    a. ultrasound
    b. CT
    c. nuclear medicine
    d. MRI

17. Graves' disease results from an excessive production of thyroid hormone known as
    a. hyperparathyroidism
    b. hyperpituitarism
    c. hyperthyroidism
    d. hypopituitarism

18. Cretinism, which usually results in short stature, is considered the result of an abnormality of an insufficient synthesis of thyroid hormone known as
    a. hypothyroidism
    b. hypopituitarism
    c. hypoparathyroidism
    d. Addison's disease

19. Thyroid adenomas appear "hot" or "cold" on nuclear medicine scans, depending on their
    a. functional capacity
    b. anatomic location
    c. interaction
    d. physiology

20. The slow-growing thyroid carcinoma with an incidence that peaks in young adulthood and in the third and fifth decades is
    a. papillary carcinoma
    b. medullary carcinoma
    c. follicular carcinoma
    d. adenocarcinoma

21. Diabetes mellitus is a result of the
    a. failure of the pancreas to secrete insulin
    b. production of excessive insulin by the pancreas
    c. conservation of water by the kidneys
    d. failure of the kidneys to conserve water

22. Sustained muscular contraction resulting from a lack of parathormone is
    a. hypothyroidism
    b. hypoparathyroidism
    c. pseudohypoparathyroidism
    d. hypopituitarism

23. The parathyroid disease process often attributed to chronic renal failure is
    a. primary hyperparathyroidism
    b. secondary hyperparathyroidism
    c. tertiary hyperparathyroidism
    d. follicular hyperparathyroidism

24. On ultrasound, which tumors generally appear as solid hypoechoic masses and may contain microcalcifications?
    a. papillary carcinomas
    b. follicular carcinomas
    c. neuroblastomas
    d. pheochromocytomas

Reproductive System

OBJECTIVES

In addition to the objectives listed at the beginning of Chapter 11 in the textbook, the user should be able to:
1. Identify anatomic structures on diagrams and radiographs of the reproductive system.
2. Describe the physiology of the reproductive system.
3. Differentiate the pathologic disorders of the reproductive system by defining the disease processes and their radiographic manifestations.
4. Determine changes in technical factors to obtain optimal-quality radiographs for patients with various underlying pathologic conditions.

EXERCISE 1: LABELING—ANATOMY

Identify the anatomic structures indicated by writing the correct names in the spaces provided.

A, The male reproductive system.

(From Solomon P: *Introduction to human anatomy and physiology*, ed 4, St. Louis, 2016, Saunders.)

B, The female reproductive system.

C, The female breast.

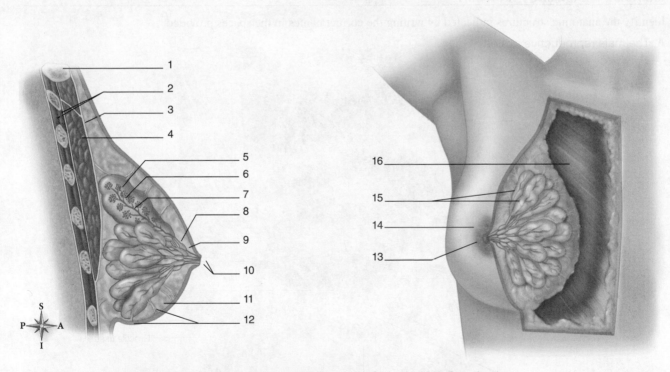

EXERCISE 2: FILL IN THE BLANK—ANATOMY AND PHYSIOLOGY

Complete the following questions by writing the correct term(s) in the blank(s) provided.

1. The major function of the male reproductive system is the _____ of _____ (spermatogenesis).

2. Male germ cells are called _____.

3. Which endocrine gland stimulates the testes to produce germ cells? _____

4. The testes produce germ cells and secrete the male hormone _____.

5. The final maturation of the sperm occurs in the _____.

6. A muscular tube that connects the epididymis and that is part of the spermatic cord is the _____.

7. The _____ _____ and the vas deferens form the ejaculatory duct.

8. Severing the vas deferens to make the male sterile is a _____.

9. The structure that lies on the posterior aspect at the base of the bladder and also secretes a thick liquid consisting of

   fructose is known as the _____ _____.

10. Male fertility depends on _____, _____, _____, and _____.

11. _____ refers to the onset of menstruation in females.

12. Ova begin to grow and develop to maturity; the process of expelling the mature ovum is known as _____.

13. The corpus luteum continues to grow after the ovum has been released and secretes _____.

14. The ovum travels from the ovary to the uterus via the _____ _____.

15. Implantation of the fertilized ovum outside of the uterus is a(n) _____ _____.

16. The _____ phase occurs between the end of menses and ovulation.

17. The phase of the menstrual cycle between ovulation and the onset of menses is _____.

18. The menstrual phase of the cycle is a result of the following three products: _____, _____,

    and _____.

19. Natural termination of the reproductive processes is _____.

20. Surgical removal of the female reproductive organs is a _____.

EXERCISE 3: FILL IN THE BLANK—REPRODUCTIVE PATHOLOGY

Complete the following questions by writing the correct term(s) in the blank(s) provided.

1. In the secondary stage of syphilis, a _____ _____ affects any part of the body.

2. _____ can cause septic arthritis (joint erosion and narrowing).

3. Radiographically, the bladder on excretory urography is elevated by a smooth impression caused by _____ _____ _____.

4. To best delineate the prostate, seminal vesicles, and surrounding organs for accurate staging of carcinoma of the prostate gland, _____ is the modality of choice.

5. Inflammation of the pair (or one) of the long, tightly coiled ducts that carry sperm from the seminiferous tubules of the testis(es) to the vas deferens is _____.

6. On ultrasound, a testicular tumor that has a uniform hypoechoic mass appearance without calcification or cystic areas is known as a _____.

7. Spread of infection into the fallopian tubes from the pelvis is caused by _____ _____ _____.

8. As a result of pelvic inflammatory disease, the fallopian tubes may be obstructed, causing _____ or _____.

9. Lipid material within the lesion with relative radiolucency that has a characteristic of calcification is a _____ _____.

10. Often multiple benign smooth-muscle tumors of the uterus, _____ _____ are stimulated by estrogen.

11. Postmenopausal bleeding is a symptom of _____ _____, which is the predominant neoplasm of the uterine body.

12. Endometrial tissue outside the uterus undergoes a proliferation and secretory phase because it responds to _____ _____.

13. The _____ _____ examination has permitted early detection of cervical carcinomas.

14. A tumor mass with clustered calcification in the mammary gland is indicative of _____ _____.

15. The most common benign breast tumor is a _____.

16. Fetal age is best demonstrated by _____.

17. Maternal disorders, such as diabetes mellitus and Rh isoimmunization, may cause _____ during pregnancy.

18. Most ectopic pregnancies occur in the _____ _____.

19. Abnormal fertilization that lacks the female chromosome is a _____.

20. Ectopic pregnancies are often associated with urine or plasma levels of _____ _____ _____ that are substantially lower for the expected date of gestation than those in patients with normal intrauterine pregnancies.

EXERCISE 4: MATCHING—ANATOMY AND PHYSIOLOGY

Match each of the following terms with the correct definition by placing the letter of the best answer in the space provided. Each question has only one correct answer. Please note that there are more terms than definitions.

1. _____ duct for ova to reach uterus

2. _____ beginning of female reproductive life

3. _____ fertilization of ova outside the uterus

4. _____ final maturation of sperm

5. _____ flow of blood, mucus, and sloughed endometrium

6. _____ formation of sperm

7. _____ male germ cells

8. _____ muscular tube passing through the inguinal canal

9. _____ time at which ova mature and are expelled from the ovary

10. _____ produces the major portion of the seminal fluid

11. _____ secrete a thick fluid of fructose

12. _____ testes secrete this male hormone

A. corpus luteum

B. ectopic pregnancy

C. ejaculatory duct

D. epididymis

E. fallopian tube

F. menarche

G. menstrual phase

H. ovulation

I. proliferative phase

J. prostate gland

K. seminal vesicles

L. spermatogenesis

M. spermatozoa

N. testosterone

O. vas deferens

EXERCISE 5: MATCHING—REPRODUCTIVE PATHOLOGY

Match each of the following terms with the correct definition by placing the letter of the best answer in the space provided. Each question has only one correct answer. Please note that there are more terms than definitions.

1. _____ arises from a primitive germ cell and consists of many tissue types

2. _____ benign ovarian tumor

3. _____ benign smooth-muscle tumor

4. _____ caused by spirochete *Treponema pallidum*

5. _____ causing an inability to empty the bladder completely

6. _____ ectopic testis

7. _____ elevated prostate-specific antigen, and a hard nodular and irregular mass on rectal examination

8. _____ excessive accumulation of amniotic fluid

9. _____ fallopian tube filled with pus

10. _____ fetal implantation outside the uterus

11. _____ fibrocystic disease—cysts of various sizes distributed throughout the organ

12. _____ follicular and corpus luteum are examples

13. _____ germ cell tumor of ovary

14. _____ infection of the uterus and fallopian tubes

15. _____ most common and most widely spread venereal disease

16. _____ most common malignancy in women

17. _____ neoplasm of the uterine body and most common invasive neoplasm

18. _____ normal-appearing endometrium in sites other than their normal location

19. _____ spectrum of pregnancy-related diseases, including hydatidiform and choriocarcinoma

20. _____ tumor arising from the seminiferous tubules

21. _____ tumor related to chronic irritation, infection, and poor hygiene

22. _____ twisting of the gonad on its pedicle

23. _____ very small volume of amniotic fluid

A. benign breast disease

B. benign prostatic hyperplasia

C. breast cancer

D. carcinoma of the prostate gland

E. cervical carcinoma

F. cryptorchidism

G. cystadenoma

H. dermoid cyst

I. ectopic pregnancy

J. endometrial carcinoma

K. endometriosis

L. epididymitis

M. fibroadenoma

N. gonorrhea

O. infertility

P. oligohydramnios

Q. ovarian cysts

R. pelvic inflammatory disease

S. polyhydramnios

T. pyosalpinx

U. seminoma

V. syphilis

W. teratoma

X. testicular torsion

Y. trophoblastic disease

Z. uterine fibroids

EXERCISE 6: MULTIPLE CHOICE

Circle the best answer for each of the following multiple choice questions.

1. On magnetic resonance imaging (MRI), benign prostatic hyperplasia appears as
   a. homogeneous low signal on T1-weighted images
   b. heterogeneous high signal on T2-weighted images
   c. normal uniform high signal intensity
   d. inhomogeneous with cystic and solid areas

2. Prostate gland carcinoma impresses on the bladder as a
   a. smooth contour with elevation
   b. irregular contour with elevation
   c. thickened bladder wall
   d. irregular contour without elevation

3. The testis normally migrates through the_____ into the scrotal sac.
   a. perineal region
   b. levator ani muscle
   c. inguinal canal
   d. cremaster muscle

4. A compromise of circulation to the testis with sudden onset of severe scrotal pain is
   a. epididymitis
   b. cryptorchidism
   c. testicular agenesis
   d. testicular torsion

5. The modality of choice to demonstrate testicular tumors is
   a. computed tomography (CT)
   b. ultrasound
   c. MRI
   d. nuclear medicine

6. Abscesses with a thick irregular wall containing echoes on pelvic ultrasound images are suggestive of
   a. pyosalpinx
   b. hydrosalpinx
   c. pelvic inflammatory disease
   d. polycystic ovarian disease

7. On an abdominal radiograph, psammomatous calcifications appearing as scattered, fine amorphous shadows (that are similar to normal soft tissue and easily missed) represent
   a. cystadenoma
   b. ovarian cyst
   c. ovarian carcinoma
   d. cystadenocarcinoma

8. A cyst (ovarian) that has no clinical significance and is composed of germ cells, such as skin, hair, and teeth, is known as a(n)
   a. polycystic ovarian disease
   b. dermoid cyst
   c. cyst adenoma
   d. ovarian cyst

9. A poorly defined mass with irregular margins and numerous fine linear strands or spicules radiating out is indicative of
   a. fibrocystic disease
   b. breast cancer
   c. benign breast disease
   d. a fibroadenoma

10. A reflux of endometrial fragments backward through the fallopian tubes during menstruation, resulting in an implantation in the pelvis, is
    a. endometriosis
    b. ectopic pregnancy
    c. trophoblastic disease
    d. pelvic inflammatory disease

11. An enlarged uterus with irregular areas of low-level echoes and bizarre clusters of high-intensity echoes is suggestive of
    a. cervical carcinoma
    b. leiomyomas
    c. ovarian cysts
    d. endometrial carcinoma

12. A benign breast disease demonstrating various-sized cysts throughout the breasts is
    a. fibrocystic disease
    b. cystoadenoma
    c. trophoblastic disease
    d. polycystic disease

13. A condition of pregnancy primarily resulting from fetal urinary disorders, such as renal dysplasia and renal aplasia, is
    a. polyhydramnios
    b. endometriosis
    c. trophoblastic disease
    d. oligohydramnios

14. An enlarged uterus that does not contain a gestational sac and that is associated with fluid in the cul-de-sac is suggestive of
    a. hydatidiform mole
    b. ectopic pregnancy
    c. choriocarcinoma
    d. endometriosis

15. Anomalies in the reproductive organs, obstructed fallopian tubes, and production of immature ova can cause
    a. pelvic inflammatory disease
    b. trophoblastic disease
    c. infertility
    d. leiomyomas

EXERCISE 7: CASE STUDY

The following is a case study in which abdominal imaging was requested. In this scenario, you will see an image and will be asked to answer questions. Using your knowledge of imaging pathology, apply exposure factors and positioning criteria to answer the questions.

CASE STUDY 1

A female patient enters the radiology department with continued symptoms of pelvic cramping. A kidney-ureter-bladder (KUB) radiograph is performed and is shown below:

1. What anatomy is a KUB required to include?

2. Technical factors should be sufficient to differentiate what anatomy?

3. Are there any abnormal structures in this image? If so, where are they located?

4. What is the differential diagnosis for this appearance?

SELF-TEST

Read each question carefully, then circle the best answer.

1. The tertiary stage of syphilis
   a. is treated with antibiotics
   b. causes multisystemic involvement
   c. results in skin lesions and a rash
   d. causes genital ulcerations

2. A bacterial infection that spreads venereal disease, causing pelvic inflammatory disease in women, is
   a. syphilis
   b. gonorrhea
   c. cytomegalovirus
   d. herpes genitalis

3. Enlargement of the prostate gland related to hormone disturbances and age is
   a. benign prostatic hyperplasia
   b. glandular carcinoma
   c. caused by an undescended testis
   d. a malignancy

4. Benign hyperplastic prostate disease causes a(n)
   a. elevated bladder with a smooth contour
   b. irregular bladder floor contour
   c. urethral stricture resulting from gonorrhea
   d. invasion of the bladder wall

5. The screening technique used to determine cryptorchidism is
   a. nuclear medicine
   b. MRI
   c. ultrasound
   d. CT

6. Absence of the testis or ectopic testis must be ruled out in cases of
   a. testicular torsion
   b. epididymitis
   c. syphilis
   d. cryptorchidism

7. Compromise of circulation and sudden onset of severe scrotal pain are suggestive of
   a. cryptorchidism
   b. epididymitis
   c. testicular torsion
   d. gonorrhea

8. Intratesticular arterial pulsations on a sonogram demonstrate good blood flow, which rules out
   a. epididymitis
   b. testicular torsion
   c. undescended testes
   d. benign prostatic hyperplasia

9. Epididymitis causes _____ on radionuclide studies.
   a. no findings
   b. a cold nodule
   c. a decreased uptake
   d. an increased uptake

10. The tumor that arises from a primitive germ cell or contains a variety of tissue is a
    a. seminoma
    b. benign hyperplasia
    c. teratoma
    d. bacterial infection

11. Normal testicular tissue is homogeneous; in cases of a seminoma, the ultrasound scan shows
    a. an inhomogeneous cystic and solid mass with calcification
    b. increased echogenicity with uniform echoes
    c. decreased echogenicity with uniform echoes
    d. a uniform hypoechoic mass without calcification

12. Metastasis from testicular tumors typically
    a. occurs at the renal hilum
    b. occurs where the gonadal veins drain
    c. is best detected by computed tomography
    d. is all of the above

13. Venereal diseases, unsterile delivery or abortion, or complications of intrauterine devices can result in
    a. polycystic ovarian syndrome
    b. dermoid cysts
    c. pelvic inflammatory disease
    d. trophoblastic disease

14. To best demonstrate pelvic abscesses, which may cause pelvic inflammatory disease, the modality of choice is
    a. CT
    b. MRI
    c. ultrasound
    d. nuclear medicine

15. Ovarian cysts appear as
    a. calcium carbonate deposits on a plain abdominal radiograph
    b. rounded anechoic adnexal masses
    c. solid irregular areas with amorphous shadows
    d. a mass with associated ascites

16. Cystic masses with several thin, well-defined septations are suggestive of a(n)
    a. cystadenoma
    b. cystadenocarcinoma
    c. ovarian cyst
    d. metastatic ovarian tumor

17. A germ cell tumor containing hair, skin, teeth, and fatty elements is
    a. a dermoid cyst
    b. an ovarian cyst
    c. polycystic ovarian disease
    d. a seminoma

18. Dermoid cysts can be demonstrated on
    a. ultrasound as anechoic masses
    b. ultrasound as hypoechoic masses
    c. radiography as radiolucencies with calcifications
    d. radiography as thickening of the bladder wall

19. A benign smooth-muscle tumor of the uterus is a
    a. fibroid
    b. cystadenoma
    c. teratoma
    d. dermoid cyst

20. The most common calcified lesion in the female genital tract is a
    a. teratoma
    b. primary cystadenocarcinoma
    c. fibroid
    d. cystadenoma

21. The invasive endometrial neoplasm of the uterine body is
    a. endometriosis
    b. endometrial carcinoma
    c. fibroid
    d. a seminoma

22. The condition in which the normal endometrium extends or appears outside the uterus is called
    a. a teratoma
    b. fibroids
    c. endometriosis
    d. pelvic inflammatory disease

23. Poor hygiene, chronic irritation, and infection appear to be related to the development of
    a. endometriosis
    b. seminomas
    c. cervical cancer
    d. ovarian cancer

24. Diffuse enlargement of the uterine body with omental metastases is indicative of
    a. leiomyomas
    b. teratomas
    c. carcinoma of the cervix
    d. endometrial carcinoma

25. In mammography, benign breast disease appears as a
    a. mass with irregular margins
    b. smooth well-circumscribed mass without extensions
    c. mass with spiculations and calcifications
    d. snowstorm because of calcifications

26. MRI is used for patients with breast implants; breast carcinoma on such images appears as a(n)
    a. hypoechoic lesion
    b. low signal intensity without spiculations
    c. high signal intensity with spiculations
    d. anechoic lesion within a thin echogenic capsule

27. In pregnancy, excessive amniotic fluid is seen in cases of
    a. oligohydramnios
    b. polyhydramnios
    c. hydramnios
    d. trophoblastic disease

28. In about half the patients with pelvic inflammatory disease, implantation of a fertilized ovum occurs in the
    a. fallopian tubes
    b. uterus
    c. vaginal canal
    d. omentum

29. The lack of a female chromosome causing an abnormal fertilization is known as a(n)
    a. choriocarcinoma
    b. hydatidiform mole
    c. seminoma
    d. ectopic pregnancy

30. _____ is a trophoblastic disease that usually appears as a large complex mass of central hemorrhage in the position at which the uterus is expected to appear.
    a. Choriocarcinoma
    b. Uterine carcinoma
    c. Teratoma
    d. Hydatidiform mole

12 Miscellaneous Diseases

12

OBJECTIVES

In addition to the objectives listed at the beginning of Chapter 12 in the textbook, the user should be able to:
1. Differentiate the pathologic disorders from the nutritional disorders and vitamin deficiencies by defining the disease processes and their radiographic manifestations.
2. Determine changes in technical factors to obtain optimal-quality radiographs for patients with various underlying pathologic conditions.
3. Describe the pathologic conditions associated with muscular dystrophy, melanoma, and systemic lupus erythematosus.
4. Differentiate hereditary abnormalities, including chromosomal aberrations and genetic amino acid disorders.

EXERCISE 1: FILL IN THE BLANK—MISCELLANEOUS PATHOLOGY

Complete the following questions regarding nutritional diseases by writing the correct term(s) in the blank(s) provided.

1. Peripheral vasodilation causes increased _____ _____, producing generalized enlargement of the cardiac silhouette.

2. The body requires _____ to complete the cellular process called respiration.

3. Weakening of capillary walls often results in bleeding into the skin, joints, and internal organs in cases of

   _____.

4. To maintain the integrity of the mucous membrane lining the respiratory, gastrointestinal, and urogenital tracts, the

   body requires vitamin _____.

5. Deposition of calcium in the kidney, heart, lungs, and stomach wall may be caused by _____.

6. Excessive eating combined with a lack of activity can result in _____.

EXERCISE 2: FILL IN THE BLANK—MISCELLANEOUS PATHOLOGY

Complete the following questions associated with the miscellaneous and hereditary diseases by writing the correct term(s) in the blank(s) provided.

1. The most frequent complaint of patients with _____ _____ _____ is pain in multiple muscles and joints.

2. Metastatic _____ also produces multiple nodules in the lung, destructive bone lesions, and hemorrhagic lesions in the brain.

3. Muscle bundles that appear finely striated or striped on radiographic images are suggestive of _____

   _____.

Chapter **12** **Miscellaneous Diseases**

4. The most common trisomy disorder of all chromosomal aberrations is _____ _____.

5. A shortened fourth metacarpal (possibly the fifth metacarpal) is a skeletal abnormality in patients afflicted with _____ _____.

6. An elongation and thinning of the tubular bones, most prominent in the hands and feet with spider-like digits, may be seen in patients with _____ _____.

7. For the body to maintain normal growth and physiologic functioning, enzymes are required to control _____ _____ metabolism.

8. Brain atrophy occurs in _____ as a result of impaired conversion of phenylalanine to tyrosine.

9. Dense laminated calcification in multiple intervertebral disks beginning in the lumbar region is seen radiographically in patients with _____.

10. Renal, urethral, and bladder stones form as a result of excessive urinary excretion of several amino acids in cases of _____.

EXERCISE 3: MATCHING—NUTRITIONAL PATHOLOGY

Match each of the following terms with the correct definition by placing the letter of the best answer in the space provided. Each question has only one correct answer. Please note that there are more terms than definitions.

1. _____ ascorbic acid deficiency

2. _____ cannot be stored and must be a regular part of the diet to prevent a deficiency

3. _____ deficiency of thiamine (vitamin B_1)

4. _____ essential for the blood-clotting mechanism to function

5. _____ excessive adipose tissue resulting from greater intake of calories than the body requires

6. _____ excessive intake of vitamin A characterized by multiple symptoms

7. _____ inability of gastrointestinal tract to digest and use proteins, carbohydrates, and lipids is one cause

8. _____ niacin deficiency

9. _____ produces abnormalities involving the gastrointestinal tract and nervous system

10. _____ results in night blindness

A. beriberi

B. hypervitaminosis

C. nutritional deficiency

D. obesity

E. pellagra

F. protein-calorie malnutrition

G. scurvy

H. vitamin A deficiency

I. vitamin D

J. vitamin K

K. vitamin K deficiency

L. water-soluble vitamins

EXERCISE 4: MATCHING—HEREDITARY PATHOLOGY

Match each of the following terms with the correct definition by placing the letter of the best answer in the space provided. Each question has only one correct answer. Please note that there are more terms than definitions.

1. _____ complex lipids accumulate in excessive amounts in the spleen, liver, and bone marrow

2. _____ connective tissue disorder affecting vision, skeletal, and cardiovascular systems

3. _____ connective tissue disorder most likely representing an immune-complex disorder

4. _____ enzyme deficiency leading to an abnormal accumulation of homogentisic acid

5. _____ error of impairment to convert phenylalanine to tyrosine

6. _____ excessive urinary excretion of several amino acids

7. _____ gonadal dysgenesis, characterized by primary amenorrhea

8. _____ group of chronic inherited conditions in which fat replaces muscle

9. _____ inborn error of the metabolism of the amino acid methionine

10. _____ malignant skin cancer

11. _____ mutation of the genes causing a disease process

12. _____ testicular dysgenesis, failure to produce sperm and testosterone

13. _____ three strands of chromosome 21 (trisomy)

A. alkaptonuria

B. arachnodactyly

C. chromosomal aberration

D. cystinuria

E. Down syndrome

F. Gaucher's disease

G. homocystinuria

H. Klinefelter's syndrome

I. kwashiorkor

J. Marfan's syndrome

K. melanoma

L. muscular dystrophy

M. Pelkan's spur

N. phenylketonuria

O. systemic lupus erythematosus

P. Turner syndrome

Circle the best answer for each of the following multiple choice questions.

1. Beriberi is caused by a deficiency of _____, resulting in a lack of growth and muscle tone.
   a. thiamine (vitamin B_1)
   b. niacin
   c. vitamin C
   d. retinol

2. The fat-soluble vitamin that is necessary to maintain the blood-clotting mechanism is
   a. vitamin D
   b. vitamin A
   c. vitamin K
   d. vitamin B_1

3. Diffuse edema, ascites, and a protuberant abdomen are clinical findings in patients with
   a. hypervitaminosis
   b. protein-calorie malnutrition
   c. obesity
   d. scurvy

4. An inborn error of amino acid transport characterized by impaired tubular absorption and excessive urinary excretion of several amino acids causing the formation of renal, ureteral, and bladder stones is
   a. cystinuria
   b. homocystinuria
   c. lupus
   d. kwashiorkor

5. Metastases from the malignant neoplasm _____ frequently involve the gastrointestinal tract as well-circumscribed, round, or oval nodules that may develop central necrosis and ulceration.
   a. sarcoidoma
   b. melanoma
   c. lupus
   d. kwashiorkor

6. Three strands of chromosome number 21 instead of the normal two result in
   a. Turner's syndrome
   b. Marfan's syndrome
   c. Klinefelter's syndrome
   d. Down syndrome

7. Testicular dysgenesis is a chromosomal aberration caused by
   a. three strands of chromosome 21
   b. an inherited generalized chromosomal disorder of connective tissue
   c. one X chromosome
   d. two or more X chromosomes

8. An error in metabolism resulting from a genetic amino acid disorder, causing a defect in the structure of collagen or elastin, is
   a. homocystinuria
   b. phenylketonuria
   c. alkaptonuria
   d. cystinuria

Read each question carefully, then circle the best answer.

1. A deficiency in what vitamin will cause vision problems due to the lack of pigment in the rods of the retina?
   a. thiamine
   b. niacin
   c. vitamin D
   d. retinol

2. The water-soluble vitamin _____ helps produce and maintain vascular endothelium.
   a. vitamin B_1
   b. vitamin B_3
   c. vitamin C
   d. vitamin D

3. In hypervitaminosis, too much calcium is absorbed from the gastrointestinal tract because of excessive
   a. vitamin B_3
   b. vitamin C
   c. vitamin D
   d. vitamin K

4. A connective tissue disorder with a characteristic butterfly-shaped rash over the nose is
   a. sarcoidosis
   b. melanoma
   c. hypervitaminosis
   d. systemic lupus erythematosus

5. Replacement of muscle by fat leads to generalized weakness and eventually causes respiratory muscle failure in
   a. muscular dystrophy
   b. multiple sclerosis
   c. sarcoidosis
   d. lupus

6. Primary amenorrhea, a result of a chromosomal aberration, is
   a. Down syndrome
   b. Turner syndrome
   c. Marfan's syndrome
   d. Klinefelter's syndrome

7. Profound retardation caused by the lack of enzyme conversion to create tyrosine occurs in infants with
   a. homocystinuria
   b. cystinuria
   c. ochronosis
   d. phenylketonuria

8. An inborn error of metabolism characterized by the accumulation of abnormal quantities of complex lipids in the reticuloendothelial cells of the spleen, liver, and bone marrow is called
   a. phenylketonuria
   b. homocystinuria
   c. gaucher disease
   d. alkaptonuria

9. A bone disease of young children in which a lack of vitamin D leads to decreased absorption of calcium from the gastrointestinal tract, resulting in weak, deformed bones is
   a. Klinefelter syndrome
   b. Rickets
   c. Tuner syndrome
   d. Marfan syndrome

10. Deposition of the black pigment of oxidized homogentisic acid in cartilage and other connective tissue causing ochronosis occurs in which disorder?
    a. cystinuria
    b. phenylketonuria
    c. homocystinuria
    d. alkaptonuria

Answer Key

CHAPTER 1

Exercise 1: Fill in the Blank

1. pathology
2. signs
3. symptoms
4. neoplasia
5. iatrogenic
6. diagnosis
7. idiopathic
8. prognosis
9. nosocomial
10. community acquired
11. inflammation
12. a. Alterations in blood flow and vascular permeability
    b. Migration of circulating white blood cells to the interstitium of the injured tissue
    c. Phagocytosis and enzymatic digestion of dead cells and tissue elements
    d. Repair of injury by regeneration of normal parenchymal cells or proliferation of granulation tissue and eventual scar formation
13. permeable
14. exudate
15. granulation
16. fibrous adhesion
17. keloid
18. a. rubor
    b. calor
    c. tumor
    d. dolor
    e. loss of function
19. heat (calor); redness (rubor)
20. exudate
21. pain (dolor); loss of function
22. pyogenic
23. suppurative
24. abscess
25. bacteremia
26. edema
27. anasarca
28. ankles; lower legs
29. lower back, sacral areas, and lungs
30. ischemia
31. infarct
32. infarctions
33. hemorrhage
34. hematoma
35. atrophy
36. hypoplasia; aplasia
37. disuse
38. Pathologic, irreversible
39. hyperplasia
40. dysplasia
41. neoplasia
42. oncology
43. benign
44. malignant
45. cancers
46. parenchyma; stroma
47. parenchymal
48. fibroma
49. adenomas
50. carcinomas
51. glandular
52. sarcomas
53. seeding; lymphatic; hematogenic
54. seeding
55. Grading; staging
56. epidemiology
57. morbidity
58. hereditary
59. Dominant; recessive
60. mutations
61. Antibodies
62. immunity
63. Vaccines; toxoid
64. acquired immunodeficiency syndrome (AIDS)

Exercise 2: Matching

1. E
2. J
3. B
4. K
5. I
6. H
7. D
8. F

Exercise 3: Matching

1. M
2. W
3. O
4. A
5. K
6. T
7. E
8. J
9. D
10. Q
11. H
12. U

13. S
14. V
15. P
16. G

17. C
18. R
19. I
20. B

Exercise 4: Multiple Choice

1. c
2. b
3. c
4. b
5. a
6. d
7. a
8. d

9. b
10. c
11. b
12. a
13. c
14. c
15. b
16. b

Self-Test

1. a
2. b
3. b
4. d
5. a
6. b
7. a
8. c
9. c
10. d
11. a
12. c
13. b

14. c
15. d
16. d
17. d
18. b
19. b
20. a
21. d
22. a
23. d
24. d
25. b

CHAPTER 2

Exercise 1: Fill in the Blank

1. imaging features or image descriptors
2. location
3. perfusion
4. FFDM, or full-field digital mammography
5. ultrasound (US)
6. Utrasound
7. computed tomography
8. computed tomography
9. magnetic resonance imaging
10. PET; positron emission tomography
11. fused *or* integrated
12. ultrasound
13. echoes
14. anechoic
15. hyperechoic, echogenic
16. isoechoic
17. patency of major blood vessels
18. direction, velocity
19. air; bone *or* barium
20. computed tomography
21. CT number
22. bone; 1000
23. lowest; air

24. 1 mm
25. spiral; helical
26. 8 to 64
27. coned x-ray, multisection
28. volume-rendered
29. maximum intensity
30. echo; repetition
31. spin-echo
32. T1-weighted
33. Cortical bone, calcium, air
34. MRI
35. Diffusion
36. fat-suppression
37. Perfusion
38. nuclear medicine (NM)
39. radiopharmaceutical
40. gamma
41. hot spot
42. single-photon emission computed tomography
43. heart; strokes
44. radiopharmaceutical; positron
45. annihilation
46. oncology; cardiology
47. integrated; direct

Exercise 2: Matching

1. U
2. I
3. L
4. Q
5. Y
6. Z
7. B
8. E
9. R
10. C

11. S
12. T
13. P
14. H
15. W
16. M
17. X
18. J
19. F
20. D

Exercise 3: Matching

1. A
2. M
3. K
4. L
5. E

6. G
7. B
8. J
9. C
10. I

Exercise 4: Multiple Choice

1. b
2. c
3. c
4. d
5. a
6. d
7. a
8. a
9. d
10. b
11. c
12. c

13. a
14. a
15. d
16. a
17. c
18. b
19. d
20. b
21. b
22. d
23. d
24. a

Self-Test

1.	d	14.	a
2.	a	15.	b
3.	c	16.	b
4.	b	17.	b
5.	c	18.	a
6.	a	19.	b
7.	b	20.	d
8.	d	21.	c
9.	b	22.	b
10.	c	23.	True
11.	e	24.	c
12.	d	25.	b
13.	a		

CHAPTER 3

Exercise 1: Labeling

A. Structure of the respiratory system:
1. cartilaginous rings
2. carina
3. left and right primary bronchi
4. secondary bronchi
5. tertiary bronchi
6. bronchiole
7. alveoli
8. capillaries
9. alveolar sac
10. alveolar duct
11. terminal bronchiole
12. hilum
13. base of lung
14. inferior lobe
15. middle lobe
16. superior lobe
17. apex
18. trachea

B. The lungs and pleura:
1. left lung
2. esophagus
3. visceral pleura
4. intrapleural space
5. pulmonary trunk
6. heart
7. sternum
8. primary bronchus
9. pulmonary vessels
10. parietal pleura
11. right lung

Exercise 2: Fill in the Blank

1. a. oxygenate blood
   b. removal of body waste
2. a. trachea
   b. bronchi
   c. bronchioles
3. conduction of air
4. mucous membrane
5. hairlike

6. Cilia
7. proliferate
8. lung parenchyma (alveoli)
9. hemoglobin; internal
10. diaphragm; intercostal; fill with air
11. body
12. visceral pleura

Exercise 3: Fill in the Blank

1. cystic fibrosis
2. Surfactant
3. epiglottitis
4. Pneumonia
5. spherical; hazy, poorly defined
6. *Mycobacterium tuberculosis*
7. coccidioidomycosis
8. Respiratory syncytial virus (RSV)
9. COPD *or* chronic pulmonary obstructive disease
10. sarcoidosis
11. silicosis
12. Bronchial adenoma
13. arteriovenous fistula

Exercise 4: Matching

1.	F	7.	L
2.	I	8.	G
3.	A	9.	H
4.	P	10.	C
5.	K	11.	B
6.	M	12.	D

Exercise 5: Matching

1.	P	12.	D
2.	L	13.	N
3.	Q	14.	F
4.	C	15.	K
5.	O	16.	G
6.	N	17.	A
7.	R	18.	V
8.	I	19.	H
9.	U	20.	S
10.	T	21.	B
11.	M		

Exercise 6: Multiple Choice

1.	b	8.	d
2.	d	9.	a
3.	a	10.	b
4.	b	11.	b
5.	b	12.	a
6.	c	13.	d
7.	b		

Exercise 7: Case Studies
Case Study 1

1. The tracheostomy tube is well visualized and placed. The tip is seen 3 to 4 cm above the carina.
2. In mobile imaging, it is common to do the image in the recumbent position, however if there is a hemorrhage, it

may be obscured. Tube placement can be determined in the recumbent image.
3. A pleural effusion or hemothorax could be obscured in the recumbent position because no fluid levels can be demonstrated.
4. A lateral decubitus position with the affected side down is needed for fluid levels, or with the affected side up for air levels.
5. There is a chest tube in the right pleural cavity.
6. The tube is to create a vacuum environment, allowing a collapsed lung to re-inflate or to remove excessive fluid in the pleural cavity.

Case Study 2

1. Not necessarily; it is difficult to see the tip of the catheter in this patient because of underexposure. The catheter appears to be in the heart because it can be seen in the superior vena cava.
2. Those viewing the image should be able to see through the heart and mediastinum. The lung markings behind the heart should be visible and the outline of the spine should be visible through the mediastinum. If not, the image is considered underexposed. If an optimal kVp (100-130) is being used, the mAs needs to be increased.
3. The tracheostomy tube is well visualized and placed. The tip is located 3 to 4 cm above the carina.
4. This would be a nasogastric (NG) tube. In this case, the patient has a tracheostomy and the oxygen is being supplemented at the ventilator. Always be sure to remove all movable tubing from the image field to reduce artifacts.
5. The three lines represent the cardiac monitoring leads (EKG). They have been straightened and moved out of the image as much as possible. By disconnecting the lines, an alarm will sound if the patient is being closely monitored. The radiographer should not remove the lines if the patient is in the intensive care unit and only when directed in other cases.

Case Study 3

1. Yes, the image contrast and density are balanced to demonstrate the tips of the leads.
2. Yes, an EKG lead is overlying the superior pacer lead, making it difficult to distinguish. The radiographer needs to move the EKG leads to the side as much as possible.
3. In the atrium near the sinoatrial (SA) node.
4. The inferior lead should be positioned at the apex of the right ventricle. It does appear in that region. A lateral projection would be required to demonstrate that the tip is directly posterior in the coronary sinus rather than in its proper position, anterior in the right ventricle.

Case Study 4

1. Yes.
2. A gastric bubble demonstrates an air-fluid level; to demonstrate it, a horizontal x-ray beam is required.
3. Increased attenuation in the right upper lobe.
4. No; consolidated material, radiopaque.
5. Yes; normal lung tissue is well demonstrated as well as the affected area.
6. Lobar pneumonia is the radiologist's differential diagnosis.

Case Study 5

1. Yes; a consolidated left lung with a mediastinal shift to the right.
2. No rotation; symmetrical sternoclavicular joints ensuring that mediastinal shift is due to pathology, not positioning error.
3. Air-fluid level in the stomach.
4. Decubitus position with a horizontal beam, affected or fluid side down; left lateral decubitus in this case. Both decubitus projections might be of benefit and may be requested.
5. Coccidioidomycosis (fungal)-pulmonary mycosis.

Self-Test

1. b	17. a
2. b	18. b
3. d	19. d
4. d	20. b
5. a	21. d
6. a	22. a
7. c	23. c
8. b	24. c
9. a	25. a
10. c	26. a
11. d	27. a
12. c	28. c
13. a	29. d
14. a	30. a
15. b	31. c
16. a	

CHAPTER 4

Exercise 1: Labeling—Anatomy

A. Long bone:
1. articular cartilage
2. spongy bone
3. red marrow cavities
4. compact bone
5. endosteum
6. medullary cavity
7. periosteum
8. epiphysis
9. diaphysis
10. epiphysis
11. Haversian system
12. osteocyte
13. spongy bone
14. compact bone
15. blood vessels
16. periosteum
B. Bone fracture and repair:
1. fracture
2. bleeding
3. bony callus
4. repaired bone

Exercise 2: Fill in the Blank—Physiology

1. bone; cartilage
2. compact bone (dense or cortical bone); cancellous bone (spongy bone)

3. outer covering—periosteum; inner lining—endosteum
4. dense; structureless
5. cancellous; spongy
6. trabeculae
7. epiphyseal
8. osteoblasts; osteoclasts
9. ossification; resorption
10. intramembranous ossification
11. osteoblasts
12. (i) supporting frame
    (ii) protects vital organs
    (iii) levers for movement
    (iv) produce blood cells in the red marrow
    (v) storage of calcium

Exercise 3: Fill in the Blank—Skeletal Pathology

1. transitional
2. spina bifida
3. achondroplasia
4. scoliosis
5. Osteoarthritis
6. Bursitis
7. osteomyelitis
8. mineralization
9. lead poisoning
10. Paget's
11. aneurysmal
12. callus
13. malunion
14. Rheumatoid arthritis

Exercise 4: Matching—Anatomy and Physiology

1. J		7. A
2. G		8. D
3. B		9. H
4. I		10. L
5. F		11. C
6. M		12. O

Exercise 5: Matching—Skeletal Pathology

1. R		12. J
2. X		13. A
3. F		14. O
4. C		15. B
5. Q		16. V
6. D		17. P
7. K		18. S
8. L		19. E
9. U		20. G
10. M		21. Y
11. I		

Exercise 6: Matching—Fracture Terms

1. F		7. A
2. C		8. G
3. D		9. N
4. K		10. B
5. M		11. J
6. I		12. E

Exercise 7: Matching—Types of Fractures

1. I		6. G
2. F		7. J
3. B		8. A
4. D		9. H
5. E		10. C

Exercise 8: Multiple Choice

1. b		8. a
2. a		9. a
3. b		10. c
4. c		11. b
5. d		12. c
6. d		13. b
7. b		14. d

Exercise 9: Case Studies

Case Study 1

1. ■ CR enters the head of the third metacarpal.
   ■ The hand is placed with the palmar surface on the image receptor so the coronal plane is parallel to the image receptor.
2. Any of the following four suggestions might be alternatives to improve the image:
   ■ Ball catcher's projection.
   ■ AP either bilateral or separately.
   ■ Do not force the patient because doing so may result in a fracture.
3. An inflammatory process.
4. Psoriatic arthritis.

Case Study 2

1. The epiphyseal growth plate proximally and distally is evidence the person is still growing.
2. Slight superimposition of the tibia and fibula both proximally and distally would indicate a true AP was completed. No, the leg is not in a true AP position. The proximal and distal tibia and fibula are too superimposed, indicating lateral rotation.
3. A radiolucency is visualized on the proximal fibula.
4. Adding the second perspective allows the radiolucency (size and location) to be more readily visualized.
5. Yes. No adjustment needed; the images demonstrate soft tissue, bony trabeculae, and cortical bone.
6. The lucency would be caused by some sort of bone erosion.
7. Bone cyst: aneurysmal or unicameral.

Case Study 3

1. The following can be seen on the dorsoplantar projection:
   ■ Artifact on the proximal shaft of the fifth metatarsal.
   ■ Tarsals are demonstrated with good bony trabeculae visible, indicating that the technique was adjusted to demonstrate this area of interest.
   ■ Toes are difficult to visualize—overexposed.
2. No, overexposed; for better visibility of detail, one of the following would be recommended:
   ■ Add a filter to attenuate a portion of the x-ray beam at the toes.
   ■ Increase the kV and lower the mAs to produce the same density and decrease the contrast.

169

3. On the oblique projection, there is a fracture of the base on the fifth metatarsal—Jones fracture.
4. The base of the fifth metatarsal is well visualized, providing a second perspective of the fracture; however, the foot is rotated. To correct this error, the radiographer should adjust the plantar surface perpendicular to the image receptor.
5. It may require two or three perspectives to demonstrate all anatomic structures without superimposition.
6. Jones fracture.

Case Study 4

1. The vertebral bodies; anterior and posterior arches of C1 are displaced.
2. Jefferson fracture, which is a comminuted fracture of the ring of the atlas involving the anterior and posterior arches with displacement.
3. If axial projections are a requirement of the protocol requested, the technologist only changed the sequence of completing the series; this is usually an acceptable practice.
4. No; the radiographer discomfort about placing the patient in hyperextension does not permit a change in orders without a physician's order—this would be outside the radiographer's scope of practice. Two alternatives are as follows:
   ■ The radiographer can speak with the radiologist and discuss the alternatives; in some cases the axial projections may be ordered.
   ■ The resident could be asked to hyperextend the patient, with monitoring for neurologic deficits; if they occur, the procedure could be stopped.

Note: In this case, it was fortunate for all parties involved that the axial images were completed first and evaluated to prevent any permanent neurologic damage.

Self-Test

1. b	13. b
2. d	14. d
3. a	15. a
4. b	16. a
5. a	17. b
6. d	18. a
7. a	19. b
8. a	20. d
9. c	21. a
10. b	22. a
11. b	23. b
12. a	24. c

CHAPTER 5

Exercise 1: Labeling—Anatomy

A. Location of the digestive organs:
  1. parotid gland
  2. pharynx
  3. esophagus
  4. liver
  5. gallbladder
  6. ascending colon
  7. ileum
  8. cecum
  9. vermiform appendix
  10. sublingual gland
  11. stomach
  12. pancreas
  13. duodenum
  14. transverse colon
  15. jejunum
  16. descending colon
  17. sigmoid colon
  18. rectum
  19. anus

B. Stomach:
  1. fundus
  2. body of stomach
  3. serosa
  4. muscularis
  5. gastric mucosa
  6. greater curvature
  7. rugae or gastric folds
  8. duodenum
  9. duodenal bulb
  10. pyloric sphincter
  11. pylorus
  12. lesser curvature
  13. lower esophageal sphincter
  14. gastroesophageal opening
  15. esophagus

C. Divisions of the large intestine:
  1. transverse colon
  2. left colic flexure
  3. descending colon
  4. sigmoid colon
  5. anus
  6. external anal sphincter muscle
  7. rectum
  8. ileum
  9. vermiform appendix
  10. cecum
  11. ileocecal valve
  12. ascending colon
  13. right colic flexure
  14. superior mesenteric artery

D. Ducts that carry bile from the liver and gallbladder:
  1. common hepatic duct
  2. common bile duct
  3. pancreas
  4. pancreatic duct
  5. sphincter muscles
  6. duodenum
  7. duodenal papilla
  8. cystic duct
  9. liver
  10. neck of gallbladder
  11. corpus (body) of gallbladder

Exercise 2: Fill in the Blank—Physiology

1. chemical; physical
2. absorbed; used
3. endocrine; exocrine
4. mouth; mastication
5. deglutition
6. chyme
7. peristalsis
8. emulsification
9. protein
10. intestinal wall
11. vitamin A; vitamin D; vitamin E; vitamin K
12. insulin; glucagon

Exercise 3: Fill in the Blank—Gastrointestinal Pathology

1. tracheoesophageal fistula
2. gastroesophageal reflux
3. corrosive agents
4. Zenker's
5. varices
6. perforation
7. pyloric stenosis
8. gastritis
9. pepsin; peptic ulcer or ulcer
10. Crohn's
11. mechanical
12. adynamic ileus
13. appendicitis
14. carcinoma
15. ulcerative colitis
16. colon cancer
17. acute cholecystitis
18. porcelain; carcinoma
19. CT
20. pathognomonic
21. perforation; ulcer
22. hepatitis
23. B

Exercise 4: Matching—Anatomy and Physiology

1. F
2. J
3. A
4. H
5. N
6. L
7. B
8. I
9. K
10. M
11. G
12. D

Exercise 5: Matching—Gastrointestinal Pathology: Esophagus and Stomach

1. K
2. O
3. H
4. J
5. P
6. R
7. M
8. A
9. B
10. N
11. F
12. Q
13. G
14. L
15. C
16. E
17. D

Exercise 6: Matching—Gastrointestinal Pathology: Small Bowel and Colon

1. D
2. N
3. E
4. A
5. I
6. G
7. F
8. O
9. H
10. B
11. J
12. P

Exercise 7: Matching—Biliary and Pancreatic Pathology

1. C
2. E
3. K
4. F
5. L
6. G
7. J
8. I
9. B
10. A

Exercise 8: Multiple Choice

1. b
2. a
3. a
4. d
5. d
6. a
7. c
8. c
9. d
10. a
11. b
12. a
13. b
14. d
15. b
16. a
17. a
18. d
19. b
20. a

Exercise 9: Case Studies
Case Study 1

1. Usually only one parent is allowed to assist because both do not need to receive radiation exposure. However, if department protocol or radiologist preference is to have the parents not assist, then the radiographer needs to communicate this information to the parents in a tactful manner. In some cases, parents are more of a hindrance than a help in getting a radiographic procedure completed.
2. The use of sterile water to dilute the barium is suggested to minimize possible infection. The amount of water required depends on the W/V concentration the radiologist requests. In infants, the concentration of barium is slightly lower than for adults.
3. A nasogastric or feeding tube has been gently placed in the pharynx so as not to cause a perforation and to visualize anatomic structures.
4. Oropharynx and laryngopharynx, which demonstrates a blunt pouch (proximal esophagus).
5. Esophageal atresia or transesophageal fistula.

Case Study 2

1. Inflammation and fibrosis cause rigid thickening of the bowel wall, resulting in a narrowing.
2. The string sign is seen in multiple areas of the small bowel.
3. Skip lesions.
4. Crohn's disease.

5. The radiologist is trying to move the barium through the small bowel and to demonstrate the diseased portion of the small bowel.
6. The formation of fistulas.

Case Study 3

1. Intussusception.
2. The coiled spring is a result of the bowel telescoping within itself (like the toy known as a Slinky).
3. The contrast/barium has moved slightly further into the colon. In this case, the radiologist externally manipulated the bowel.
4. The enema bag should run by gravity flow being approximately 24 inches above the table. To ensure that perforation will not occur from increased pressure as a result of the enema.
5. The intussusception has been relieved; the bowel is now fully filled.
6. Both; diagnostic in demonstrating the pathologic condition and therapeutic in relieving the telescoping bowel.
The infant was relieved of the intussusception upon completion of the barium enema; however, the intussusception relapsed the following day and surgery had to be performed.

Case Study 4

1. Air-fluid level in the stomach.
2. It is recommended that the patient be in the upright position for a minimum of 5 minutes (10 to 20 minutes is preferred) to allow air-fluid levels to form.
3. Place the patient into the required position before completing any other procedural criteria. When the remaining steps are completed, enough time will have passed that the image will demonstrate air-fluid levels.
4. Any and all upright images should be completed first to ensure air-fluid levels. In this case, the patient already has air-fluid levels from sitting; doing the upright imaging first is more efficient in this case.
5. Yes; under both diaphragms. There is air pushing down the stomach and liver.
6. Pneumoperitoneum.
7. A left lateral decubitus projection.

Self-Test

1. c	15. b
2. a	16. a
3. b	17. b
4. d	18. d
5. a	19. b
6. c	20. c
7. c	21. a
8. d	22. c
9. a	23. a
10. d	24. b
11. b	25. b
12. d	26. a
13. b	27. c
14. c	

CHAPTER 6

Exercise 1: Labeling—Anatomy

A. Location of the urinary system:
1. renal artery
2. renal vein
3. left kidney
4. abdominal aorta
5. inferior vena cava
6. urethra
7. urinary bladder
8. ureter
9. right kidney
10. liver
11. adrenal gland

B. Internal structure of the kidney:
1. fibrous capsule
2. cortex
3. minor calyces
4. major calyces
5. medullary pyramid
6. medulla
7. ureter
8. renal papilla of pyramid
9. renal pelvis
10. hilum
11. renal sinus

C. Structure and location of the male urinary bladder:
1. peritoneum (cut away)
2. smooth muscle
3. trigone
4. ureteral opening (L)
5. internal urinary sphincter
6. urethra
7. external urinary sphincter
8. prostate gland
9. rugae
10. ureteral opening (R)

Exercise 2: Fill in the Blank—Anatomy and Physiology

1. waste products; reabsorb; secrete
2. nephron
3. glomerulus
4. proximal convoluted tubule
5. descending limb; loop; ascending limb
6. electrolyte; acid-base
7. papillae
8. renal pelvis
9. reservoir
10. right ureter; left ureter; urethra
11. trigone
12. void; micturate
13. urethra
14. sphincter muscles
15. incontinence

Exercise 3: Fill in the Blank—Urinary Pathology

1. compensatory hypertrophy
2. malrotated
3. ureterocele
4. duplication
5. horseshoe kidney
6. glomerulonephritis
7. tuberculosis
8. papillary necrosis
9. kidney stones
10. staghorn
11. hydroureter
12. ureteropelvic junction; ureterovesical junction; bladder neck; urethral meatus
13. renal cyst
14. polycystic kidney
15. hematuria; flank pain; possibly palpable abdominal mass
16. renal carcinoma
17. Wilms' tumor
18. carcinoma
19. Renal vein thrombosis
20. Acute renal failure

Exercise 4: Matching—Anatomy and Physiology

1. F
2. N
3. H
4. B
5. M
6. J
7. O
8. I
9. D
10. E
11. G
12. C

Exercise 5: Matching—Urinary Pathology

1. T
2. R
3. S
4. I
5. G
6. H
7. K
8. N
9. Q
10. B
11. P
12. D
13. E
14. U
15. F
16. O
17. J
18. M
19. C
20. L

Exercise 6: Multiple Choice

1. b
2. a
3. b
4. a
5. a
6. a
7. b
8. d
9. a
10. d
11. c
12. a
13. d
14. b
15. d
16. c
17. c
18. c

Exercise 7: Case Studies

Case Study 1

1. On the left, there is a radiolucent line on the posterior aspect of the contrast-enhanced kidney. Posterior to the kidney, blood representing a hematoma is seen as an area more radiolucent than the opaque contrast-enhanced kidney.
2. Yes; the blood does not enhance and the kidney does because of the vascularity of the kidney.
3. Kidney fracture with a hematoma.
4. A hematoma or bleeding from the trauma.
5. Right kidney; contrast-enhanced kidney parenchyma and renal pelvis are anterior to the mass. The kidney has lost the smooth contour because of the hematoma.
6. Large renal hematoma on the right, positioned posterior to the kidney.

Case Study 2

1. To demonstrate the bowel preparation in scheduled cases; if any pathology is evident before the contrast injection, it will be visualized.
2. In the left kidney tissue (cortex or parenchyma), there is evidence of a renal calculus (radiopaque).
3. If there is a blockage, drainage will be reduced, causing the kidney to remain contrast-enhanced for a longer period. The renal calculus may be obscured by the contrast agent because of similar attenuation factors in the contrast agent and the stone.
4. There are two radiopaque objects in the area of the bladder.
5. No; the objects will be obscured by the contrast agent.
6. Stones in the bladder lodged in diverticula.

Phleboliths are a possibility on the initial image; the radiographs must demonstrate that the stones are in the bladder.

Case Study 3

1. Foley catheter, which is used to fill the bladder in the retrograde approach.
2. An early bladder image to ensure that the bladder is filling without complication.
3. The bladder outline is normal for the patient's age; on the inferior right, there is an extension of the bladder that is questionable.
4. Extends inferiorly through a "neck" on the right side.
5. Whether the lesion was located anteriorly or posteriorly in reference to the bladder. In this case, the filling defect is anteriorly located.
6. There is a filling defect inferior to the bladder with connection; questionable fistula or herniation.

Differential radiologic diagnosis: 16 cm × 9 cm mass in the right scrotum, which is compatible with a bladder herniation or large diverticulum projecting through the inguinal canal in the right side of the scrotum.

Self-Test

1. c
2. b
3. a
4. a
5. c
6. b
7. b
8. c
9. d
10. a
11. c
12. a
13. c
14. b
15. a
16. d
17. a
18. b
19. a
20. b

173

CHAPTER 7

Exercise 1: Labeling—Anatomy

A. Conduction system of the heart and vascular anatomy:
1. aortic arch
2. pulmonary artery
3. pulmonary veins
4. mitral (bicuspid) valve
5. Purkinje fibers
6. left ventricle
7. bundle of His
8. inferior vena cava
9. right ventricle
10. tricuspid valve
11. right atrium
12. atrioventricular (AV) node
13. pulmonary veins
14. sinoatrial (SA) node
15. superior vena cava

B. Structure of the heart valves:
1. left atrioventricular valve or mitral valve (open)
2. pulmonary semilunar valve (open on C, closed on B)
3. aortic semilunar valve (open on C, closed on B)
4. left atrioventricular valve or mitral valve (closed)
5. right atrioventricular valve or tricuspid valve (open)
6. right atrioventricular valve or tricuspid valve (closed)

C. Principal arteries:
1. left common carotid artery
2. left jugular vein
3. left subclavian vein
4. aortic arch
5. left pulmonary artery
6. pulmonary trunk
7. left pulmonary vein
8. celiac artery
9. left renal artery
10. abdominal aorta
11. left common iliac artery
12. left internal iliac artery
13. left external iliac artery
14. left femoral artery
15. right femoral vein
16. right common iliac vein
17. inferior vena cava
18. right renal vein
19. hepatic vein
20. right pulmonary vein
21. right pulmonary artery
22. right axillary artery
23. superior vena cava
24. right subclavian artery
25. right jugular vein
26. right common carotid artery

Exercise 2: Fill in the Blank—Anatomy and Physiology

1. supply; blood
2. rhythmic contractions
3. autonomic
4. Epinephrine
5. right atria; right ventricle; left atria; left ventricle
6. regurgitation *or* backflow
7. smooth muscle
8. cusps; right; right
9. ventricles; heart
10. Systemic
11. Pulmonary
12. Systemic; left
13. diastole
14. SA node; AV node

Exercise 3: Fill in the Blank—Cardiovascular Pathology

1. ventricular septal defect
2. Patent ductus arteriosus
3. high ventricular septal defect; overriding of the aortic orifice above the ventricular defect; pulmonary stenosis; right ventricular hypertrophy
4. Coarctation
5. fatty
6. myocardial infarction
7. left
8. dilate *or* open
9. cardiac enlargement; redistribution of pulmonary venous flow; interstitial and alveolar edema; pleural effusion
10. increasing SID; performing AP versus PA projections; recumbent versus upright positioning
11. cardiothoracic (C/T)
12. pulmonary venous
13. pulmonary edema
14. cardiac output; total peripheral resistance
15. saccular; fusiform
16. calcification
17. massive hemorrhage
18. right displacement of nasogastric tube; widening of the right paratracheal stripe; apical pleura cap sign
19. thrombus
20. Echocardiography

Exercise 4: Matching—Anatomy and Physiology

1. A
2. D
3. J
4. N
5. I
6. C
7. F
8. P
9. O
10. M
11. K
12. L

Exercise 5: Matching—Cardiovascular Pathology

1. S
2. Q
3. C
4. V
5. O
6. W
7. B
8. R
9. F
10. L
11. H
12. K
13. U
14. I
15. G
16. D
17. J
18. A
19. E
20. P

Exercise 6: Multiple Choice

1. a	11. c
2. c	12. a
3. a	13. d
4. a	14. d
5. c	15. d
6. d	16. a
7. d	17. c
8. b	18. a
9. d	19. b
10. a	20. a

Exercise 7: Case Studies

Case Study 1

1. For this AP image, the patient was erect; the labeling was provided by the technologist who produced the image.
2. The heart may appear enlarged as a result of the AP positioning; however, the image is marked as such so the radiologist can account for this change. The heart is a greater distance from the IR, creating OID = magnification. Yes, the radiologist will realize the change because the image has been labeled with the difference.
3. Decreased SID; do we know what SID was used? Recumbent versus erect; the heart will appear larger in a recumbent image.
4. Cardiomegaly; congestive heart failure.
5. The size of the patient's fist on an upright image. No; it is enlarged laterally in both directions.
6. Cardiothoracic ratio; the heart should be less than 50% of the thoracic cavity width.

Case Study 2

1. No.
2. Calcium deposits, which are common in the aorta and sometimes seen in the iliac and carotid arteries.
3. Yes; calcium (bone) is radiopaque, described on a KUB radiograph as a linear calcification outlining the aortic wall.
4. Enlarged, or greater than normal.
5. Pelvis.
6. The iliac arteries.
7. Yes; on the left in the iliac artery. The aneurysm extends into the iliac arteries.

Self-Test

1. d	16. b
2. b	17. a
3. c	18. c
4. a	19. b
5. d	20. d
6. a	21. c
7. a	22. a
8. d	23. b
9. d	24. a
10. a	25. b
11. c	26. c
12. b	27. b
13. b	28. a
14. c	29. c
15. a	30. a

CHAPTER 8

Exercise 1: Labeling—Anatomy

A. Structure of a neuron:
1. dendrite
2. cell body
3. nucleus
4. axon
5. synaptic terminal branches
6. myelin sheath

B. Divisions of the brain:
1. cerebrum
2. corpus callosum
3. cerebellum
4. brainstem
5. medulla oblongata
6. pons
7. midbrain
8. hypothalamus
9. pineal body
10. thalamus
11. diencephalon

C. Coverings and structures of the central nervous system:
1. white matter
2. gray matter
3. spinal nerve
4. dura mater
5. arachnoid
6. pia mater
7. autonomic (sympathetic) ganglion
8. spinal cord
9. dura mater
10. arachnoid
11. pia mater
12. ventral/dorsal root

Exercise 2: Fill in the Blank—Anatomy and Physiology

1. peripheral nervous [system] (PNS)
2. Afferent
3. central nervous system (CNS); peripheral effectors
4. autonomic
5. neuron
6. axon
7. myelin sheath
8. synapse
9. reflux arc
10. motor; efferent
11. cortex
12. cerebrum
13. gyri
14. White
15. sensory; motor
16. Visual
17. opposite
18. corpus callosum
19. basal ganglia
20. brainstem
21. cerebellum

22. cranial bones *or* skull
23. pia mater; arachnoid membrane; dura mater
24. aqueduct; Sylvius
25. foramen; Monro
26. lateral
27. tentorium cerebelli
28. thalamus
29. central nervous system; peripheral nervous system
30. third ventricle; thalamus; hypothalamus

Exercise 3: Fill in the Blank—Nervous System Pathology

1. viral meningitis
2. meningitis
3. encephalitis
4. *Haemophilus influenzae;* pneumococci; meningococci
5. brain abscess
6. MRI
7. epidural
8. subdural empyema
9. diastatic
10. depressed
11. subdural; epidural; intracerebral
12. biconvex
13. subdural
14. cerebral contusions
15. subarachnoid hemorrhage
16. fracture
17. blowout; CT
18. zygomatic arch
19. tripod
20. mandible
21. nasal bones
22. cerebrovascular disease
23. rule out; exclude
24. TIA *or* transient ischemic attack
25. duplex color *or* Doppler
26. intraparenchymal

Exercise 4: Fill in the Blank—Nervous System Pathology

1. MRI
2. neoplasm *or* tumor
3. acoustic neuroma
4. chromophobe adenoma
5. Craniopharyngiomas
6. germinomas; teratomas
7. chordoma
8. metastatic carcinoma
9. Petit mal
10. PET
11. normal aging
12. stooped posture; stiff and slow movement; fixed facial expression; involuntary rhythmic limb tremor
13. Huntington's
14. noncommunicating; normal-pressure
15. sinusitis

Exercise 5: Matching—Anatomy

1. H		6. G
2. F		7. D
3. I		8. K
4. E		9. C
5. L		10. J

Exercise 6: Matching—Neuroanatomy

1. C		10. P
2. E		11. I
3. W		12. G
4. H		13. Z
5. D		14. M
6. Q		15. X
7. N		16. T
8. B		17. S
9. F		18. K

Exercise 7: Matching—Nervous System Pathology

1. I		11. Q
2. H		12. A
3. F		13. S
4. M		14. E
5. L		15. D
6. B		16. O
7. C		17. J
8. T		18. P
9. U		19. R
10. K		20. G

Exercise 8: Matching—Nervous System Pathology

1. O		10. L
2. F		11. J
3. G		12. H
4. S		13. B
5. I		14. Q
6. M		15. D
7. A		16. N
8. K		17. T
9. R		18. C

Exercise 9: Multiple Choice

1. a		11. a
2. d		12. a
3. b		13. c
4. c		14. b
5. d		15. c
6. a		16. a
7. c		17. d
8. b		18. d
9. a		19. a
10. c		20. b

Exercise 10: Case Studies
Case Study 1

1. Left upper hilar region.
2. Conventional tomography, CT, MRI.

3. The greater the arc (40 degrees), the thinner the slice. Exposure time must be adequate to expose the image receptor during the full arc to produce the thinnest slice.
4. Abscess; in this case the cause was tuberculosis.
5. A ring of contrast enhancement outlining the abscess capsule.

Case Study 2

1. Carotid.
2. Carotid endarterectomy.
3. Aneurysm.

Case Study 3

1. Cerebrovascular malformation.
2. The vessels that were feeding the region were occluded or blocked.

Case Study 4

1. Cerebrospinal fluid.
2. Hydrocephalus; noncommunicating and normal-pressure.
3. Ventricular shunt to drain the CSF to the abdominal peritoneum or the cardiovascular system.
4. CT to determine the ventricular and sulcus size and MRI for the disorder causing the obstruction.

Self-Test

1. c	11. b
2. a	12. b
3. c	13. d
4. a	14. a
5. c	15. b
6. b	16. a
7. b	17. d
8. a	18. b
9. b	19. c
10. b	20. d

CHAPTER 9

Exercise 1: Labeling

1. red blood cells (erythrocytes)
2. platelets (thrombocytes)
3. white blood cells (leukocytes)
4. granular leukocytes
5. basophil
6. neutrophil
7. eosinophil
8. nongranular leukocytes
9. lymphocyte
10. monocyte

Exercise 2: Fill in the Blank—Anatomy and Physiology

1. oxygen; nutrients; salts; hormones
2. infection; toxic substances; foreign antigens
3. red bone marrow; lymph nodes
4. erythrocytes (red blood cells); thrombocytes (platelets); leukocytes (white blood cells)
5. red bone marrow; lymphoid tissue

6. (i) neutrophils (55%-75%)
   (ii) eosinophils (1%-4%)
   (iii) basophil (up to 1%)
   (iv) lymphocyte (25%-40%)
   (v) monocytes (2%-8%)
7. neutrophil
8. platelet

Exercise 3: Fill in the Blank—Hematopoietic Pathology

1. anemia
2. spherocytosis; sickle cell anemia; thalassemia
3. sickle cell
4. thalassemia
5. Megaloblastic
6. secondary polycythemia
7. myelocytic leukemia
8. lymphatic leukemia
9. leukemia
10. lymphomas
11. lymph nodes; spleen; lymphoid tissue of parenchymal organs
12. Hodgkin's disease
13. lymph nodes
14. non-Hodgkin's lymphoma
15. mediastinum
16. PET (positron emission tomography)
17. mononucleosis
18. platelets; calcium; 12 co-enzymes and proteins
19. Purpura

Exercise 4: Matching—Anatomy and Physiology

1. F		5. J	
2. E		6. D	
3. H		7. K	
4. A		8. B	

Exercise 5: Matching—Hematopoietic Pathology

1. D	7. A
2. N	8. H
3. B	9. M
4. G	10. E
5. K	11. C
6. F	12. L

Exercise 6: Multiple Choice

1. c	6. b
2. b	7. d
3. a	8. a
4. a	9. d
5. a	10. c

Exercise 7: Case Study

Case Study 1

1. Hodgkin's lymphoma usually originates in the lymph nodes, whereas in non-Hodgkin's lymphoma, the parenchymal organs are involved (approximately 40% are extranodal).

2. CT to rule out retroperitoneal adenopathy in the chest, abdomen, and pelvis. MRI and PET to demonstrate lymphomatous involvement of the abdomen and pelvic nodes. US to detect abdominal retroperitoneal adenopathy. PET to demonstrate microscopic tumor foci and altered function in normal-size nodes.
3. Transversely, 8.9 cm; AP diameter, 10.4 cm.
4. Region 1 = CT number 60; Region 2 = CT number 85; Region 3 = CT number −101.
5. Region 1.
6. Region 3.

Self-Test

1. b	6. c
2. b	7. a
3. c	8. a
4. d	9. b
5. a	10. a

CHAPTER 10

Exercise 1: Labeling—Anatomy and Physiology

A. Adrenal gland:
  1. adrenal gland
  2. kidney
  3. capsule
  4. cortex
  5. medulla
B. Pituitary and hormones:
  1. antidiuretic hormone (ADH)
  2. oxytocin (OT)
  3. growth hormone (GH)
  4. prolactin
  5. gonadotropic hormones (FSH and LH)
  6. thyroid-stimulating hormone (TSH)
  7. adrenocorticotropic hormone (ACTH)
C. Thyroid and parathyroid glands:
  1. hyoid bone
  2. larynx
  3. superior parathyroid gland
  4. thyroid gland
  5. isthmus
  6. inferior parathyroid glands
  7. trachea

Exercise 2: Fill in the Blank—Anatomy and Physiology

1. adrenal gland
2. Mineralocorticoids
3. carbohydrate metabolism
4. masculinize the body; retain amino acids; enhance protein synthesis
5. epinephrine; norepinephrine
6. hypothalamus
7. sella turcica
8. body; development
9. posterior; smooth muscle
10. thyroxine
11. thyroid gland
12. parathyroid glands
13. increased calcium absorption; prevents loss of calcium; secretes calcitonin
14. Diabetes mellitus

Exercise 3: Fill in the Blank—Endocrine System Pathology

1. Cushing's syndrome
2. aldosteronism
3. adrenogenital
4. adrenal
5. biochemical tests
6. neuroblastomas
7. hyperpituitarism
8. gigantism
9. Hypopituitarism
10. diabetes insipidus
11. nuclear medicine (radionuclide scanning)
12. benign thyroid adenoma
13. papillary; follicular; medullary
14. primary; secondary; tertiary
15. Diabetes mellitus

Exercise 4: Matching—Anatomy and Physiology

1. P	9. E
2. J	10. I
3. M	11. L
4. R	12. C
5. A	13. B
6. Q	14. D
7. O	15. N
8. G	

Exercise 5: Matching—Endocrine System Pathology

1. I	11. M
2. G	12. H
3. E	13. R
4. F	14. C
5. J	15. D
6. N	16. W
7. O	17. K
8. U	18. B
9. V	19. P
10. S	20. T

Exercise 6: Multiple Choice

1. c	9. b
2. a	10. b
3. d	11. a
4. a	12. a
5. b	13. b
6. b	14. a
7. b	15. c
8. d	

Self-Test

1. d	5. d
2. a	6. a
3. b	7. a
4. a	8. c

9. b	17. c
10. b	18. a
11. b	19. a
12. c	20. a
13. c	21. a
14. c	22. b
15. d	23. b
16. c	24. a

CHAPTER 11

Exercise 1: Labeling—Anatomy

A. The male reproductive system:
1. urinary bladder
2. vas deferens
3. urethra
4. spermatic cord
5. penis
6. testis
7. glans penis
8. scrotum
9. epididymis
10. bulbourethral gland
11. prostate gland
12. ejaculatory duct
13. seminal vesicle

B. The female reproductive system:
1. isthmus of uterine tube
2. ovarian ligament
3. ampulla of uterine tube
4. infundibulum of uterine tube
5. infundibulopelvic ligament
6. fimbriae
7. broad ligament
8. uterine artery and vein
9. vagina
10. external os of vaginal cervix
11. fornix of vagina
12. cervix of uterus
13. cervical canal
14. internal os of cervix
15. myometrium
16. endometrium
17. uterine body cavity
18. body of uterus
19. fundus of uterus

C. The female breast:
1. clavicle
2. intercostal muscle
3. fascia of pectoral muscles
4. pectoralis major muscle
5. alveolus
6. ductule
7. duct
8. lactiferous duct
9. lactiferous sinus
10. nipple pores
11. adipose tissue
12. suspensory ligaments of Cooper

13. nipple
14. areola
15. alveoli
16. pectoralis major muscle

Exercise 2: Fill in the Blank—Anatomy and Physiology

1. formation; sperm
2. spermatozoa
3. anterior lobe of the pituitary gland
4. testosterone
5. epididymis
6. vas deferens
7. seminal vesicle
8. vasectomy
9. seminal vesicles
10. number of sperm; size of sperm; shape of sperm; motility of sperm
11. Menarche
12. ovulation
13. progesterone
14. fallopian tubes (uterine)
15. ectopic pregnancy
16. proliferative (postmenstrual)
17. secretory (postovulation)
18. blood; mucus; sloughed endometrium
19. menopause
20. hysterectomy

Exercise 3: Fill in the Blank—Reproductive Pathology

1. nonitching rash
2. Gonorrhea
3. benign prostatic hyperplasia
4. MRI
5. epididymitis
6. seminoma
7. pelvic inflammatory disease
8. infertility; ectopic pregnancy
9. dermoid cyst
10. uterine fibroids
11. endometrial carcinoma
12. hormonal changes
13. Papanicolaou smear
14. breast cancer
15. fibroadenoma
16. ultrasound
17. polyhydramnios
18. fallopian tubes
19. hydatidiform mole
20. human chorionic gonadotropin (HCG)

Exercise 4: Matching—Anatomy and Physiology

1. E	7. M
2. F	8. O
3. B	9. H
4. D	10. J
5. G	11. K
6. L	12. N

179

Exercise 5: Matching—Reproductive Pathology

1. W	13. H
2. G	14. R
3. Z	15. N
4. V	16. C
5. B	17. J
6. F	18. K
7. D	19. Y
8. S	20. U
9. T	21. E
10. I	22. X
11. A	23. P
12. Q	

Exercise 6: Multiple Choice

1. a	9. b
2. b	10. a
3. c	11. d
4. d	12. a
5. b	13. d
6. c	14. b
7. d	15. c
8. b	

Exercise 7: Case Study

Case Study

1. Kidneys, ureters, and bladder. The superior symphysis pubis should be included.
2. Lateral abdominal wall, properitoneal fat layer (flank stripe), psoas muscles, lower border of the liver, and kidneys, inferior ribs, and transverse processes of the lumbar vertebrae.
3. Yes; in the right pelvis inlet/outlet, radiolucencies look like teeth.
4. Dermoid cyst.

Self-Test

1. b	16. a
2. b	17. a
3. a	18. c
4. a	19. a
5. c	20. c
6. d	21. b
7. c	22. c
8. b	23. c
9. d	24. c
10. c	25. b
11. d	26. c
12. d	27. b
13. c	28. a
14. c	29. b
15. b	30. a

CHAPTER 12

Exercise 1: Fill in the Blank—Miscellaneous Pathology

1. cardiac output
2. niacin (or vitamin B3)
3. scurvy
4. A
5. hypervitaminosis
6. obesity

Exercise 2: Fill in the Blank—Miscellaneous Pathology

1. systemic lupus erythematosus
2. melanoma
3. muscular dystrophy
4. Down syndrome
5. Turner syndrome
6. Marfan's syndrome
7. amino acid
8. phenylketonuria
9. alkaptonuria
10. cystinuria

Exercise 3: Matching—Nutritional Pathology

1. G	6. B
2. L	7. C
3. A	8. E
4. J	9. F
5. D	10. H

Exercise 4: Matching—Hereditary Pathology

1. F	8. L
2. J	9. G
3. O	10. K
4. A	11. C
5. N	12. H
6. D	13. E
7. P	

Exercise 5: Multiple Choice

1. a	5. b
2. c	6. d
3. b	7. d
4. a	8. a

Self-Test

1. d	6. b
2. c	7. d
3. c	8. c
4. d	9. b
5. a	10. d